AF876635

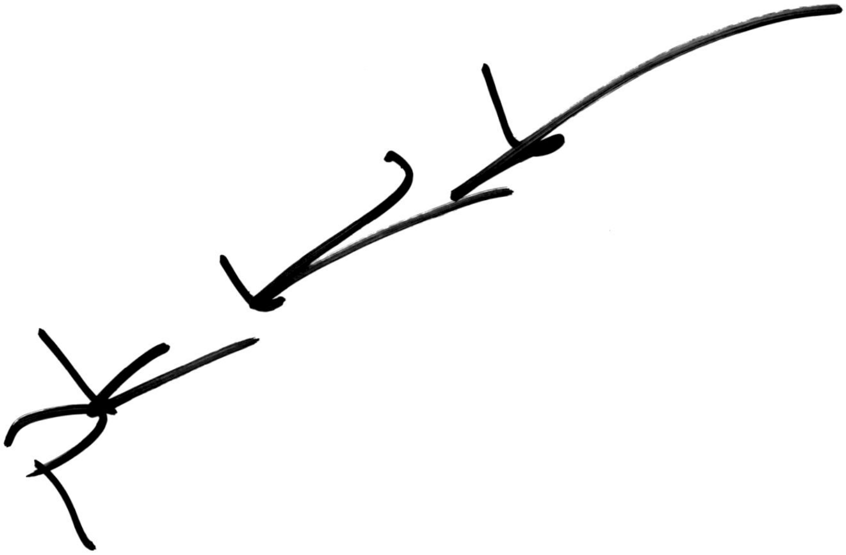

# SILENT GLORY

**images of a FIRE/EMS department**

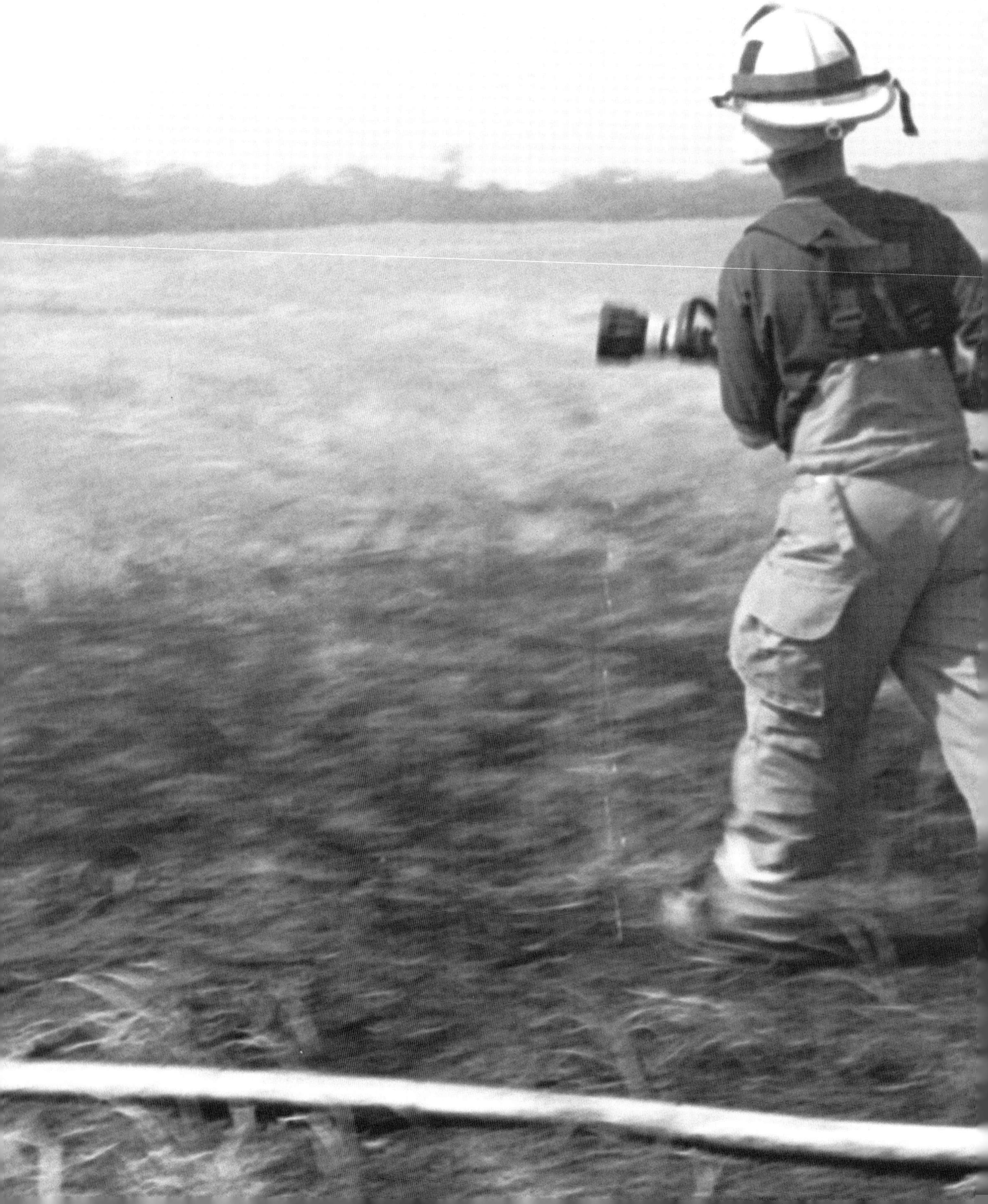

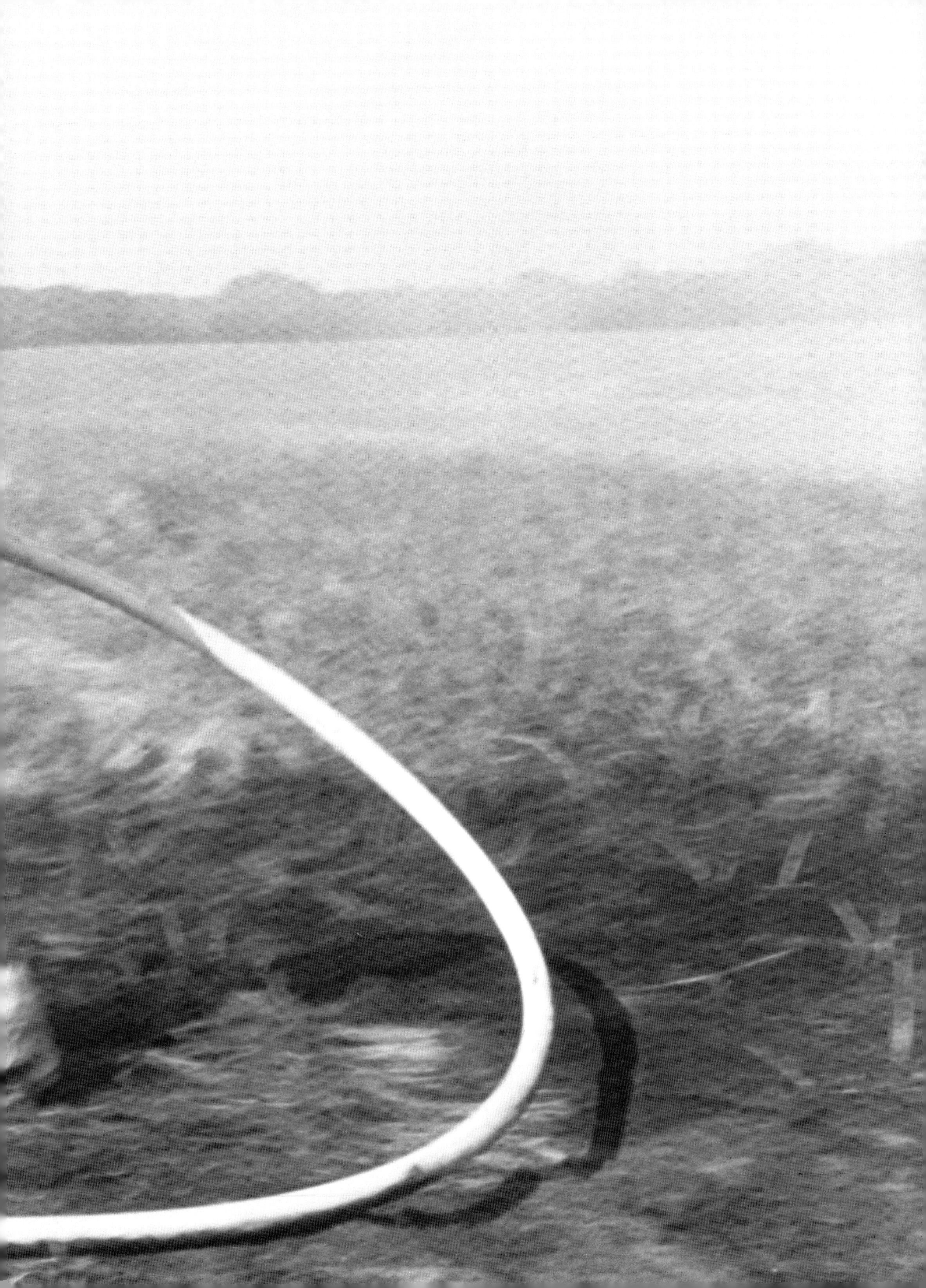

# SILENT GLORY

**images of a FIRE/EMS department**

Photographs by Pete Knudsen

Foreword by Frank Roma
Assistant Fire Chief
McKinney, Texas

pb publishing (a service of esense corporation-tx)

# SILENT GLORY

**images of a FIRE/EMS department**

by Peter K. Knudsen

Published by:
pb publishing
(a service of esense corporation)
Box 9
Weston, Texas 75097-0009
Web site: esensecorp.us
e-mail: writeus@esensecorp.us



P-CIP:

Knudsen, Peter K.
Silent glory : images of a fire/EMS department / photographs by Peter K. Knudsen ; foreword by Frank Roma. -- 1st ed.
p. cm.
ISBN 0-9721779-0-6

1. Fire departments--Texas--McKinney--Pictorial works. 2. Emergency medical services--Texas--McKinney--Pictorial works. I. Title.

TH9505.M35K68 2002 363.37'09764556
QBI02-200577

International Bookland bar code: 9 780972 1777900 53995
ISBN: 0-9721779-0-6
SAN: 254-6620

# Table of contents

# Foreword

There is much to be said for being in the right place at the right time. And so it was, that I was in that "right place at the right time" one afternoon back in June 2001. A tentative knock on my office door followed by the appearance of a man I did not know but offered a friendly smile and asked for just a moment of my time to talk about the possibility of taking some pictures of a community Fire Department. Pete Knudsen introduced himself as a photography student who was working on a documentary project as part of his course of study at the local Collin County Community College.

His assignment was to submit six photographs that would become part of a larger permanent collection which was archiving elements and aspects of life in Collin County. He thought a local Fire Department would make an interesting subject for his project; and I thought there would be no better Fire Department than ours.

We talked a bit about the legal and safety issues involved in riding out with our engine companies and the unique culture of the Fire Service in general. Pete was given 24 hour carte-blanche to all our stations, equipment and most importantly our Firefighters.

For Pete's project to be truly effective, I knew that he would have to establish a relationship with those he wished to photograph and spending time at our stations and with our members could only do that. What I did not know was that "Picture Pete" as we all affectionately know him, was interested in EVERYTHING!

If it was in our stations or on our trucks, if we wore it to fight fires or treat the sick and injured, Pete saw an opportunity for a picture. He rode with us to fires, accidents, medical calls and public education events. He ate with us and slept at our stations. He came to know our families. You name it, and he was there. And being there, he saw things from a perspective different than that of our own or the public.

The images in this book capture that perspective which not only honors the photographer, but the photographed as well. Pete became a part of our "Family" and as such, was with us as we experienced the horror of 9-11. He was able to feel both the pain and concern of our members as we processed those events. He was able to gain an understanding into the bond and brotherhood that exists among all Firefighters as we mourned for the 343 lost with the FDNY. He was also able to see the resolve and commitment of our members as we pondered the possibilities of what the future might hold for us in the post 9-11 world and our role in it on the front lines of the Homeland Defense.

What started as a project to take just a few photographs in a few weeks turned into thousands of images taken over nearly a year. Pete often told me how honored he felt to be able to be given an insiders view of our world, the world of a Firefighter and the life within a typical community fire department. But it was his sense of humor and humility that allowed him to become a part of us. In December 2001, we honored Pete at our departmental awards banquet with the rank of "Honorary Deputy Chief".

We are proud of the work Pete has done profiling the men, women, and work of our Fire Department, and thank him for being our friend.

I hope that through his photographs, which graphically tell our story, you may also have a sense of pride in the work that Firefighters perform not only here, but all across our country and throughout the world.

Frank Roma
Assistant Fire Chief
McKinney Fire Department
McKinney, Texas

# Dedication

This book is gratefully dedicated to
Firefighters who selflessly risk their lives to
provide emergency medical care,
fire suppression and prevention
for all people and property
throughout the world.

# Introduction

**Silent Glory** contains representative images from an on-going photo-documentary project to preserve "life as we know it at the turn of the millennium" for future generations. I selected today's Firefighters as my subject for 2001. Little did I know at the start that the work would evolve into this book, or that my timing would be fitting, considering the fateful day of 9/11.

McKinney Texas Fire Chief Mark Wallace and Assistant Fire Chief Frank Roma were key to the success of the project through their immediate approval, encouragement and continued support. Their leadership spirit of "let's roll" is also the essence of all their Firefighters. From day one, I was "family" which made the experience an unbelieveable journey.

I hope the images represent much more than an isolated moment and say something far greater than an incidental story. I trust they begin to unfold the larger dimension and demonstrate the universal character that is the quiet satisfaction and honor of all Firefighters everywhere, at home and abroad.

They put it on the line for us every day, with hardly our notice or second thought. We seem to forget how they selflessly put themselves in harm' way for us, driven by their honor, spirit and devotion to serve. I trust this book will remind us all of their dedicated work and their personal sacrifices on our behalf.

Many thanks to Chiefs Wallace and Roma, the shift Battalion Chiefs, Station Captains, Fire Marshal, dispatch team, administrative staff and in particular the men and women Firefighters who made this project possible, memorable and hopefully, a lasting tribute to all those who serve their neighbors. Their story... their glory.

The project was well underway for more than three months when the tragedies of 9-11 occurred. The terrorist attacks which killed so many Firefighters brought new meaning and recognition of their work to me. Your local community Firefighters battle the same terror of fires, medical emergencies and a score of other dangerous and life threatening situations that will endanger some of us, our families, and our property, every day. God bless them all...

Pete Knudsen
Weston, Texas

# fire

Silent Glory is not of fires, rather the Firefighters, and their selfless courage and honor.

Destructive fire is neither glamorous nor noble. The same is said of war. But through the chaos of both emerge those we respect and hold in grateful appreciation for their gallantry and bravery. We revere the warrior and their strife, not the battleground or theater.

The following photographs are images of real fires, real drama, and very real Firefighters. Nothing was staged or contrived. The pictures may not be the dazzling images of the "towering infernos" of our larger cities, but the circumstances are just as devastating and destructive, just as terrifying and perilous for those in the struggle.

The Firefighters of your community fire department are in similar situations somewhere in your town every day, every night. Their very personal Silent Glory is having the opportunity to serve their fellow citizens by selflessly protecting their neighbors lives, loved ones and property from the ravages of fire and medical crisis. These photographs both represent and raise tribute to them.

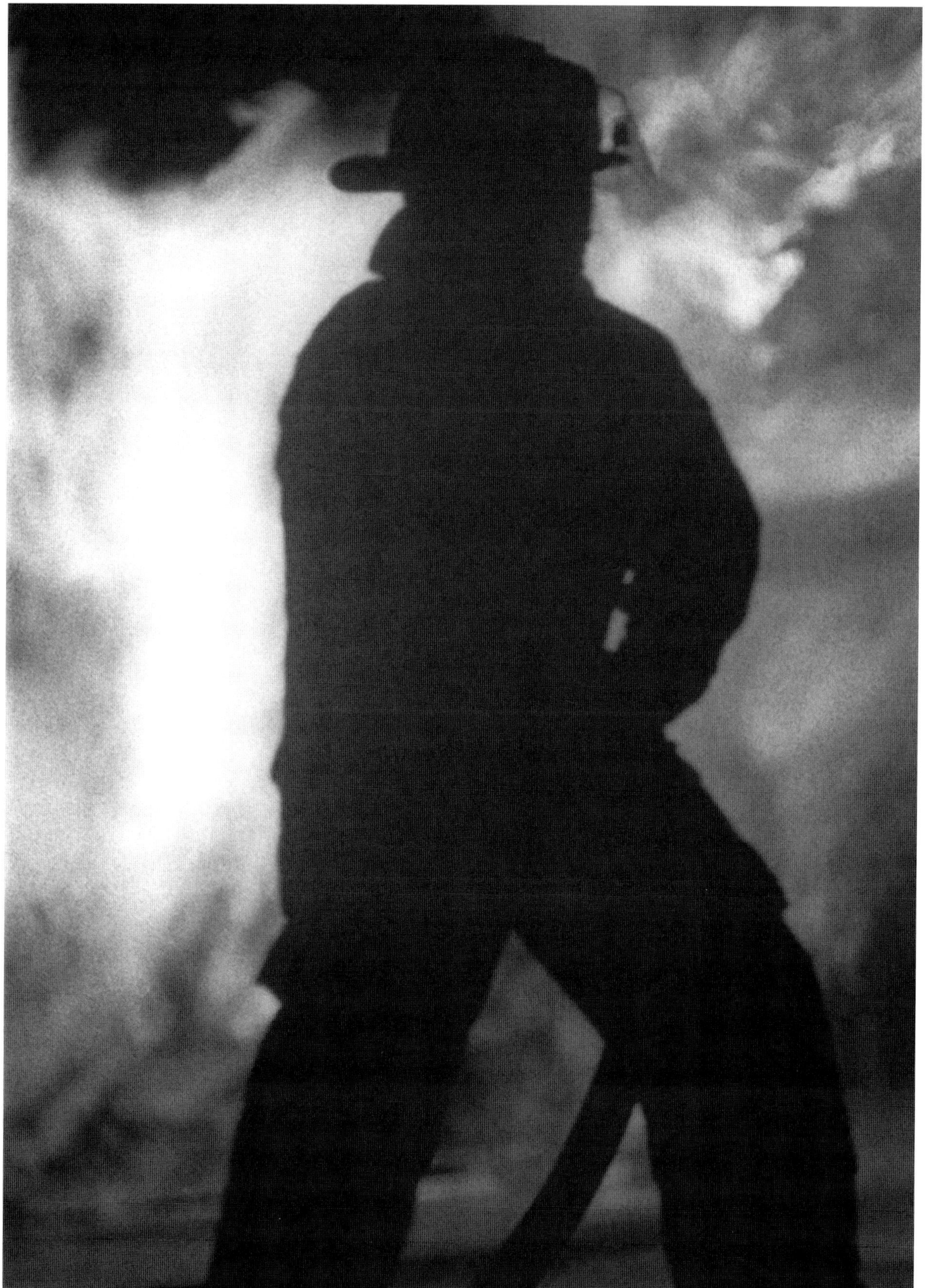

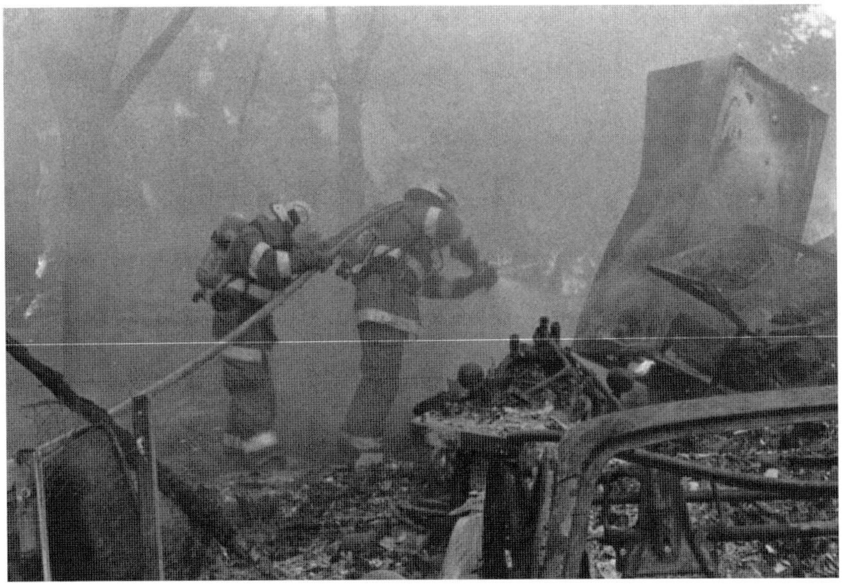

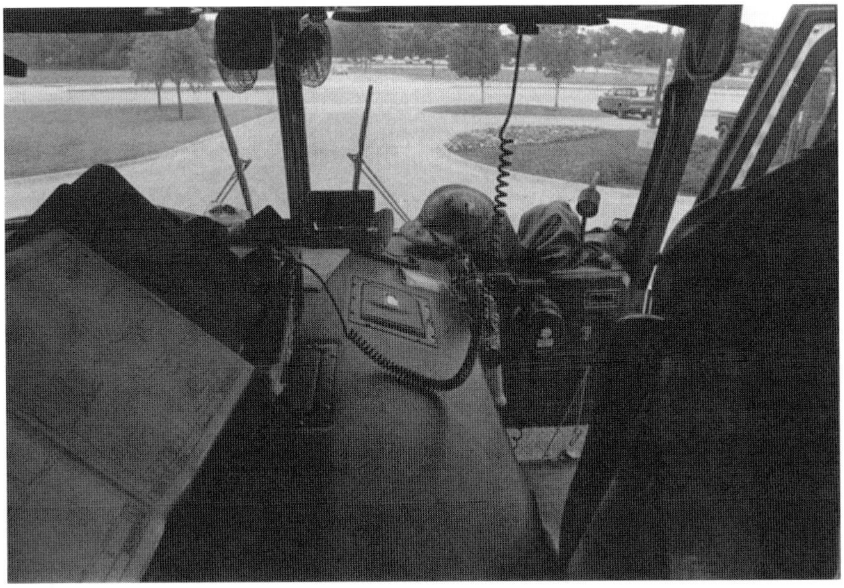

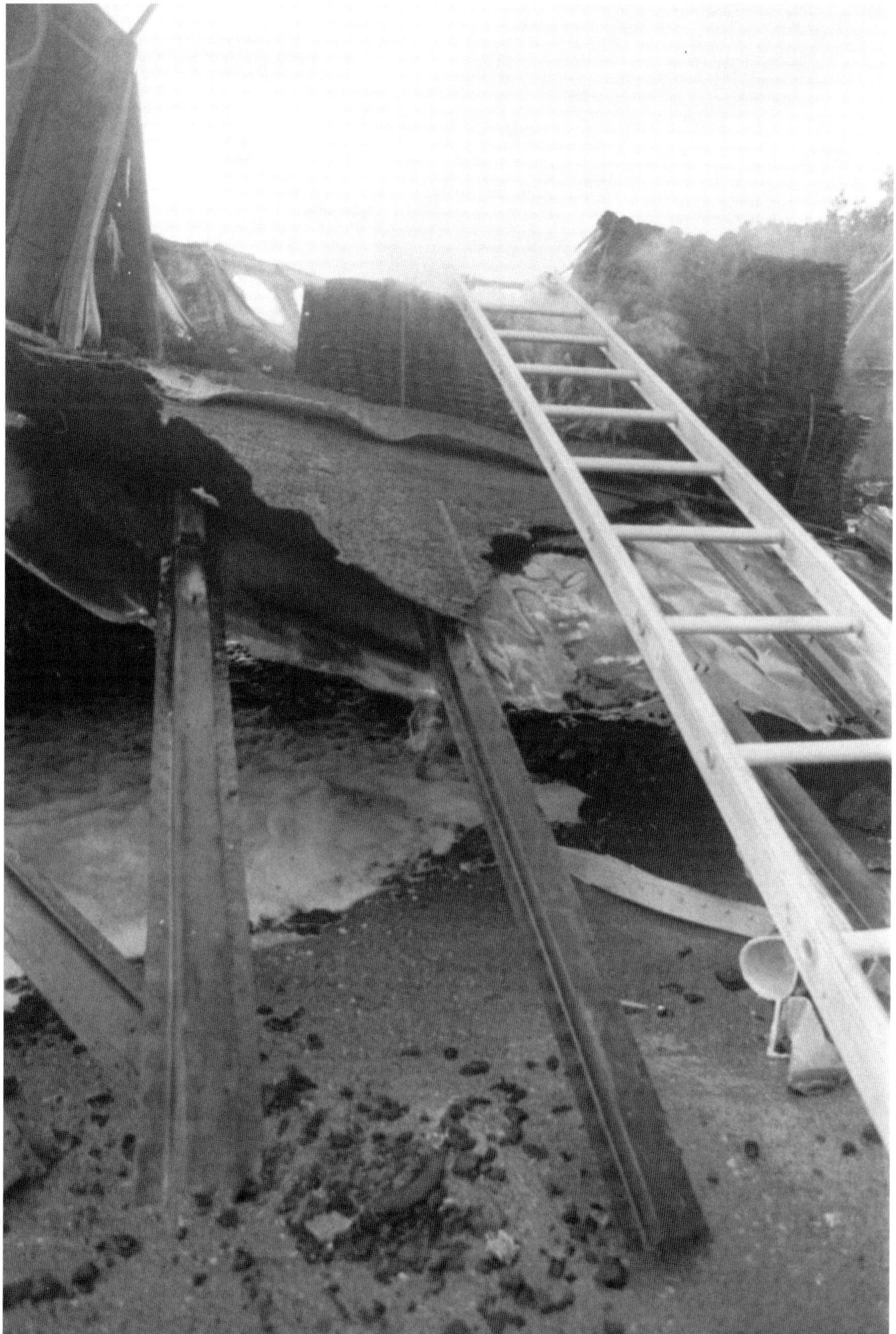

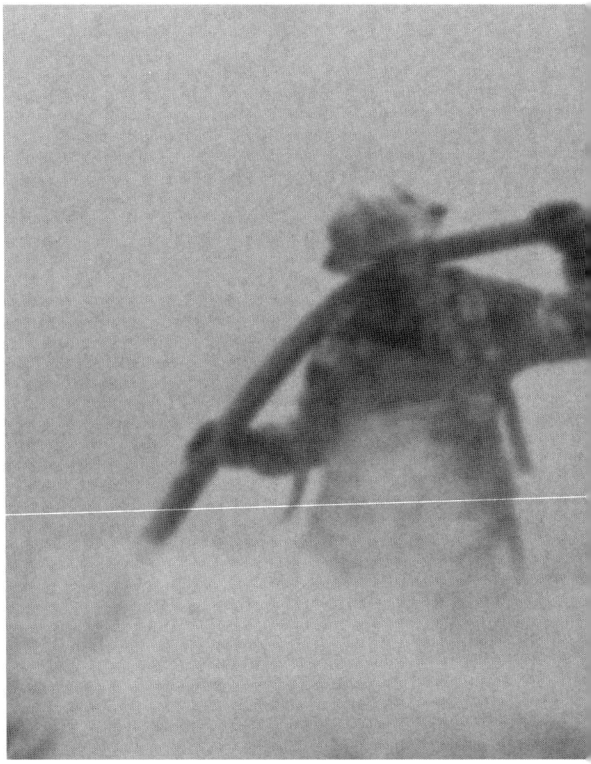

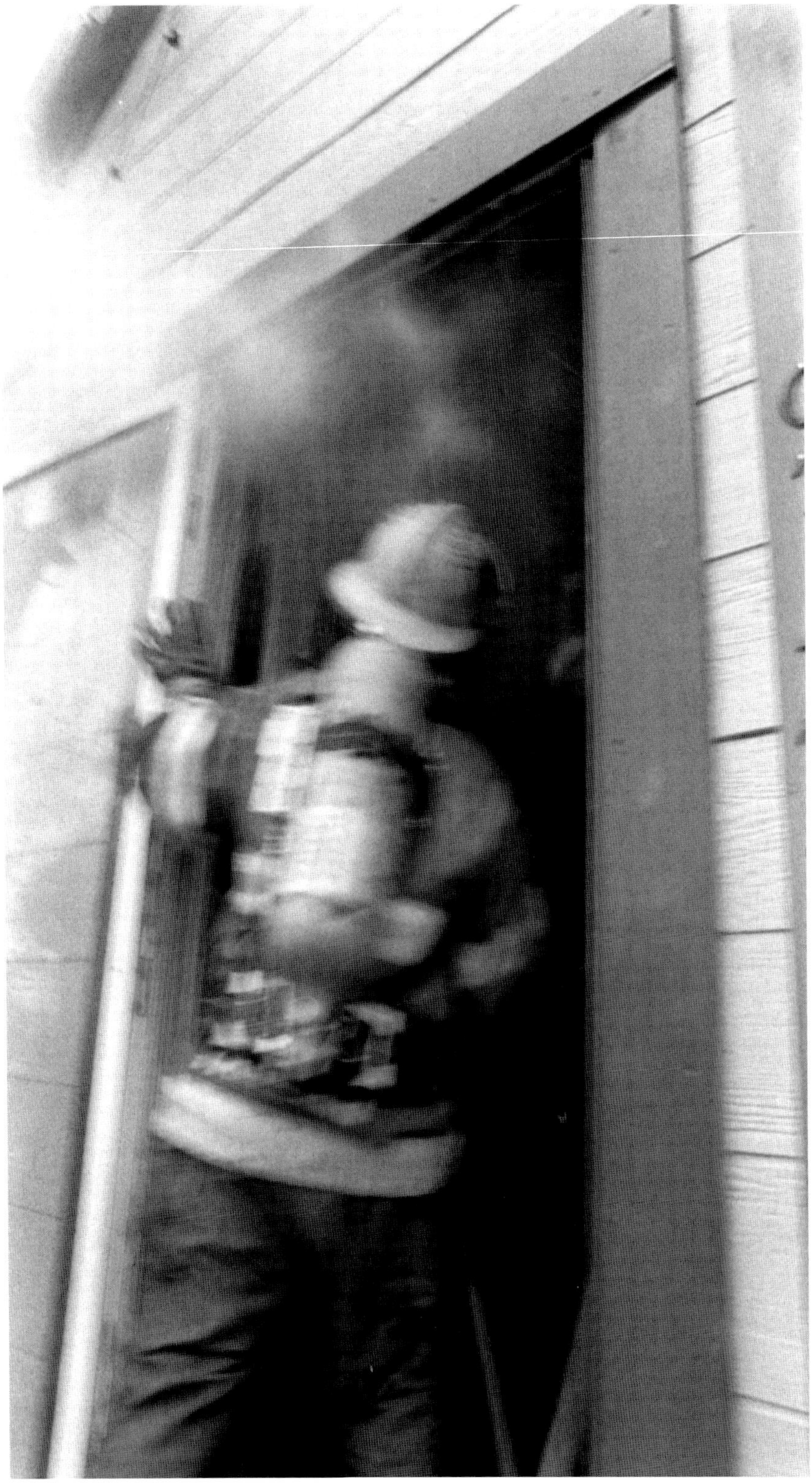

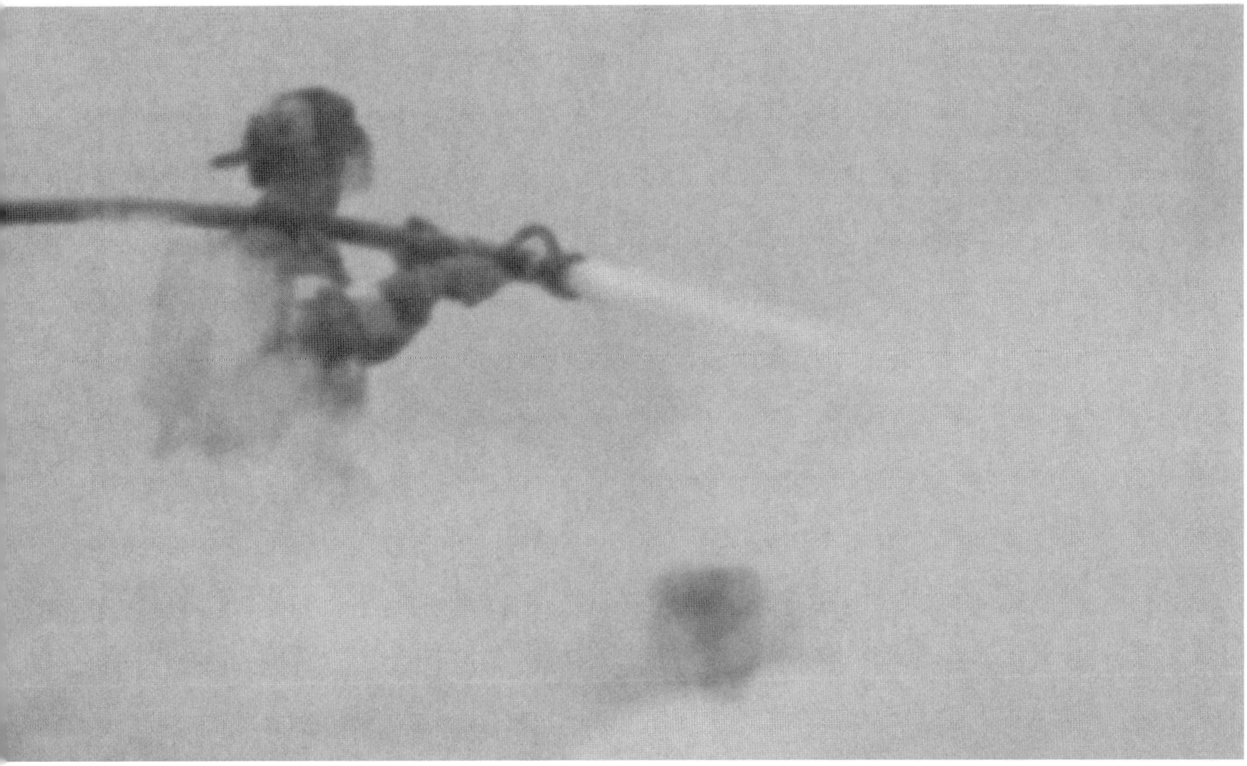

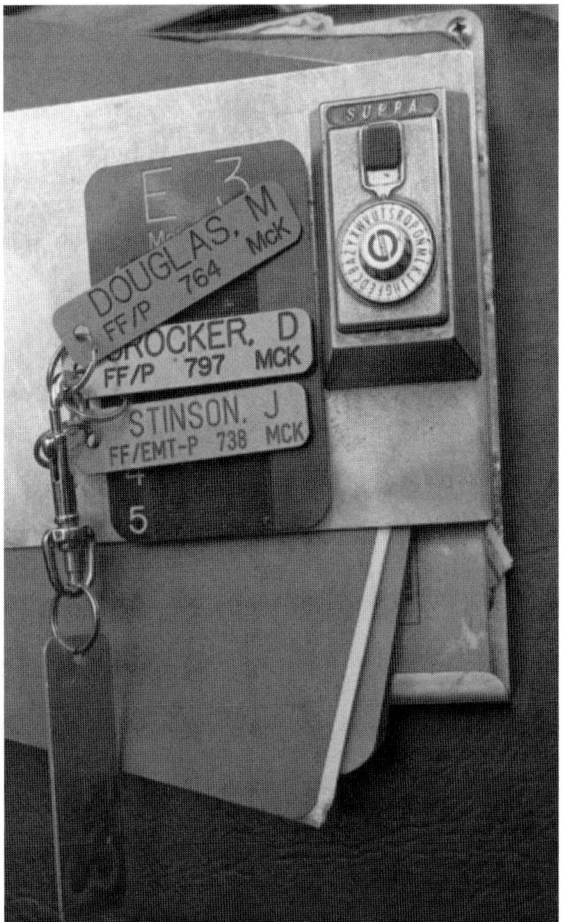
SUPRA
E 3
DOUGLAS, M
FF/P 764 McK
FF/P 797 MCK
STINSON, J
FF/EMT-P 738 MCK
5

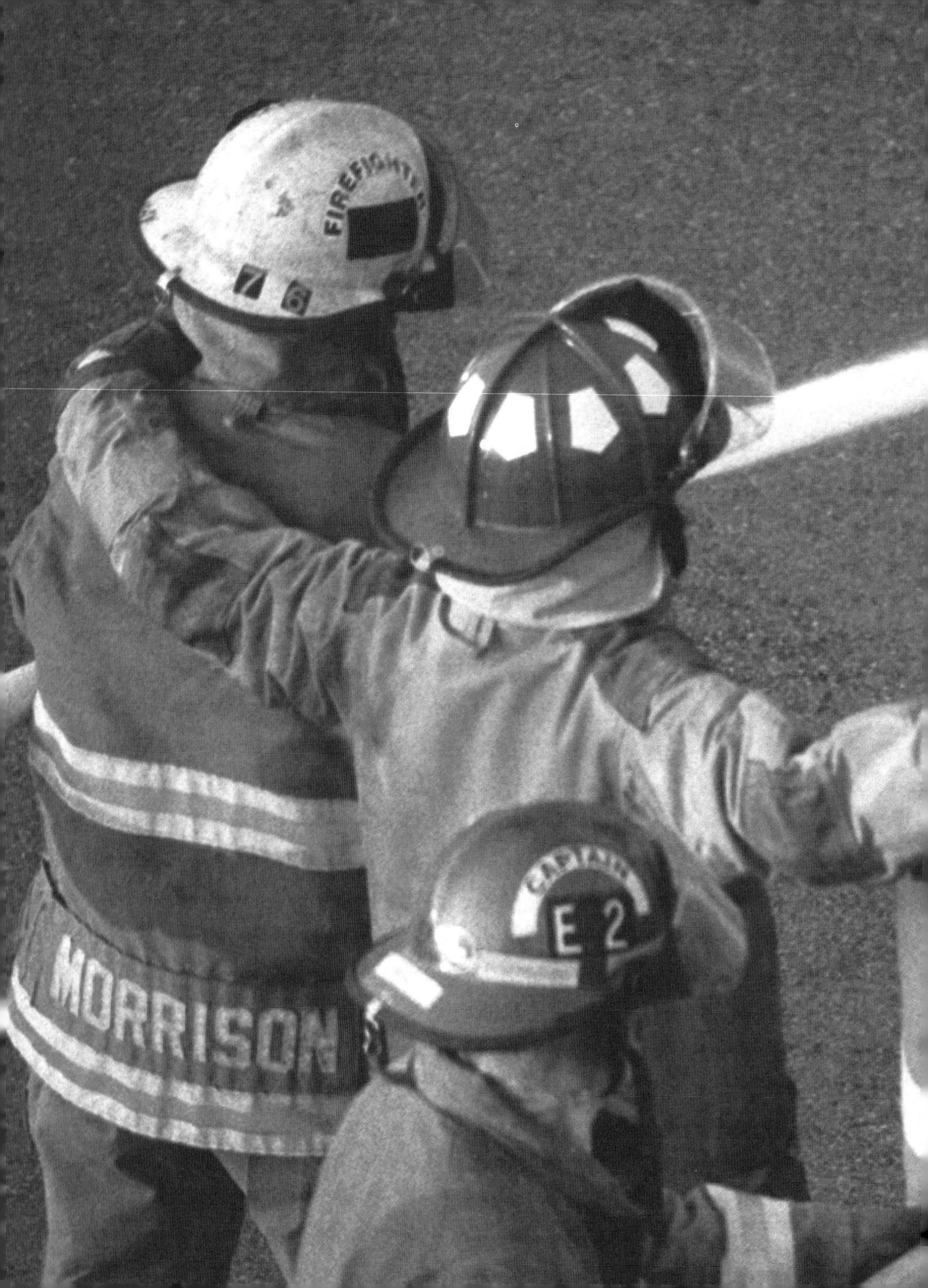
76
E 2
MORRISON

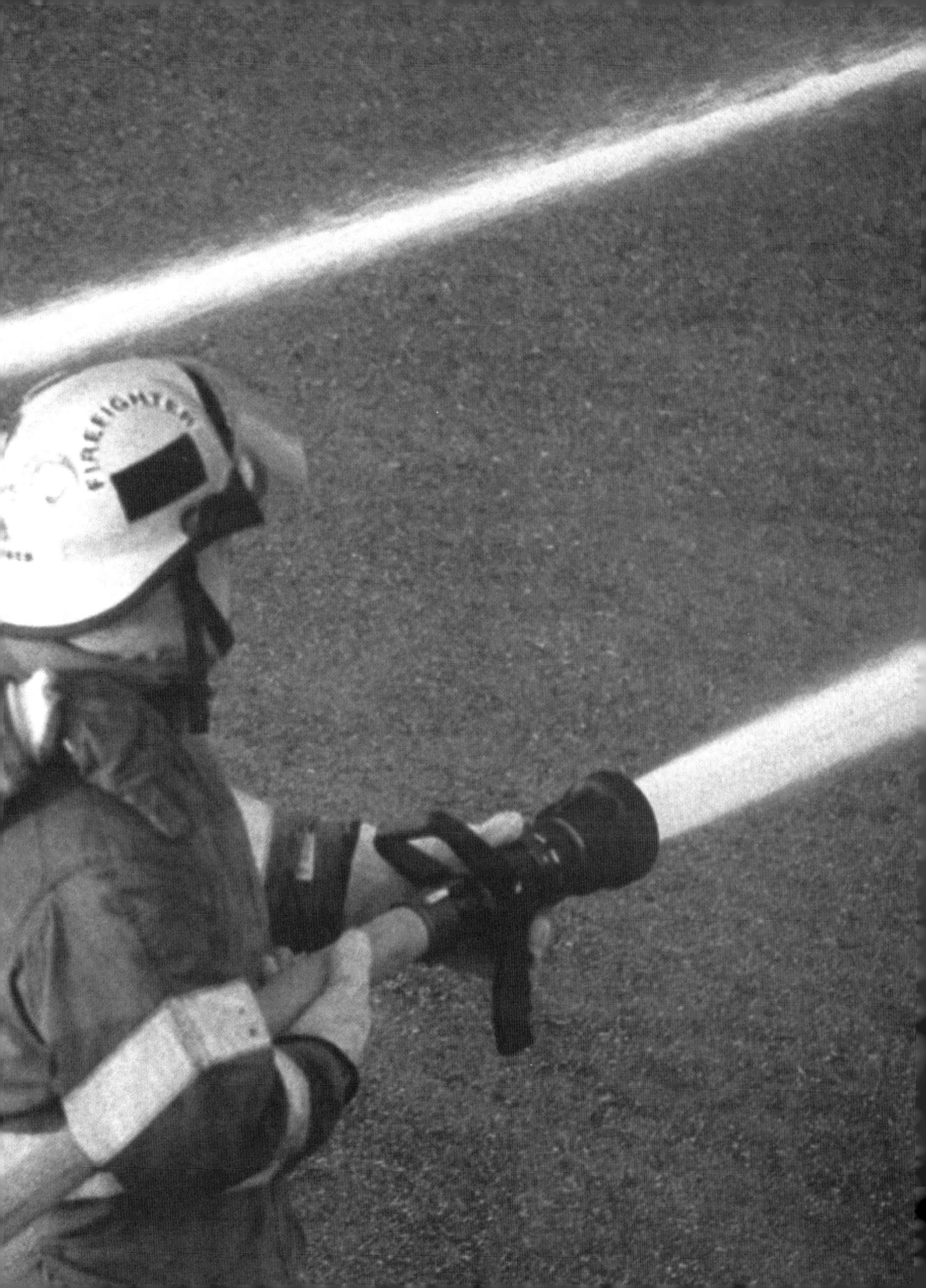
FIREFIGHTER

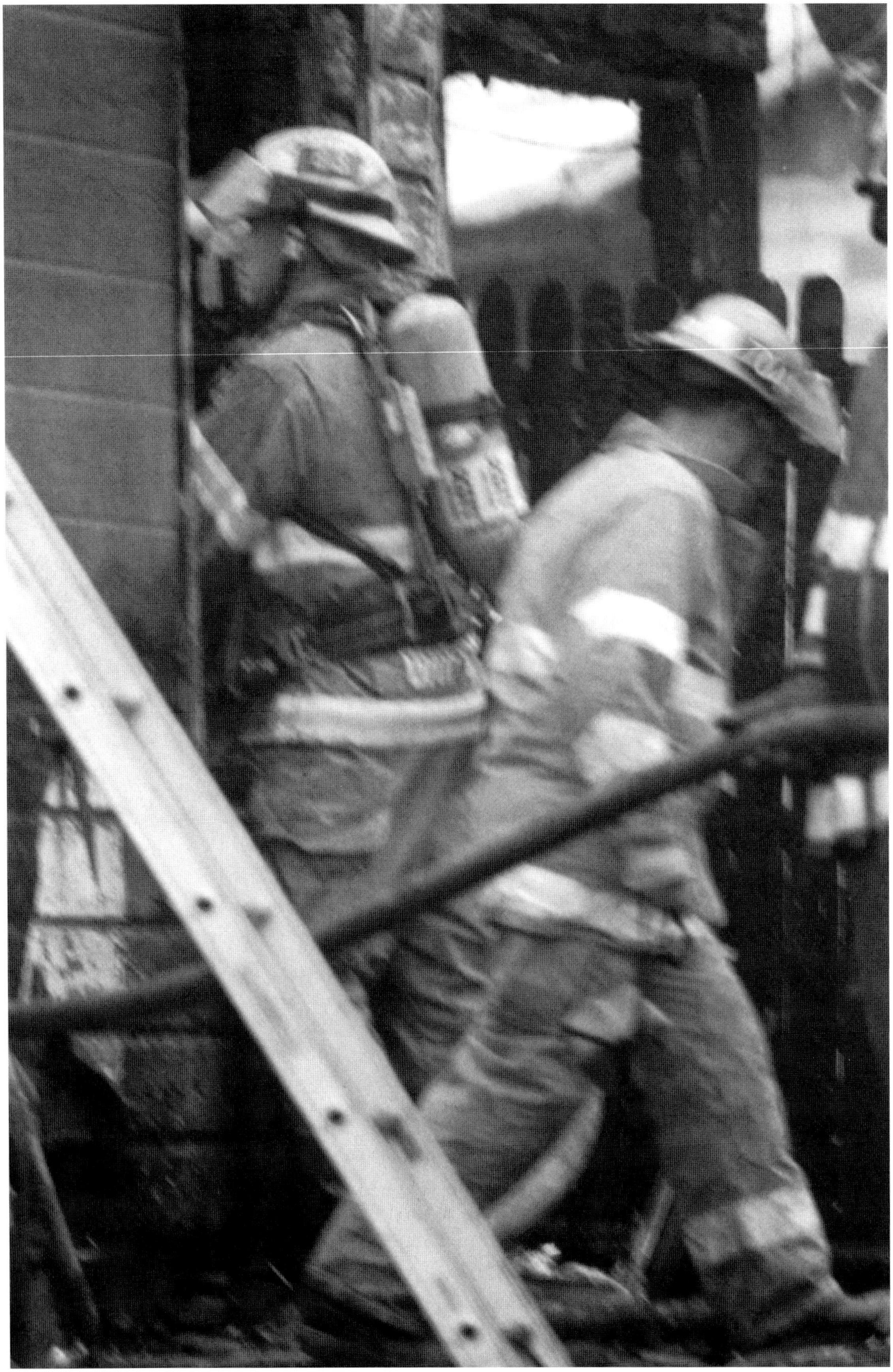

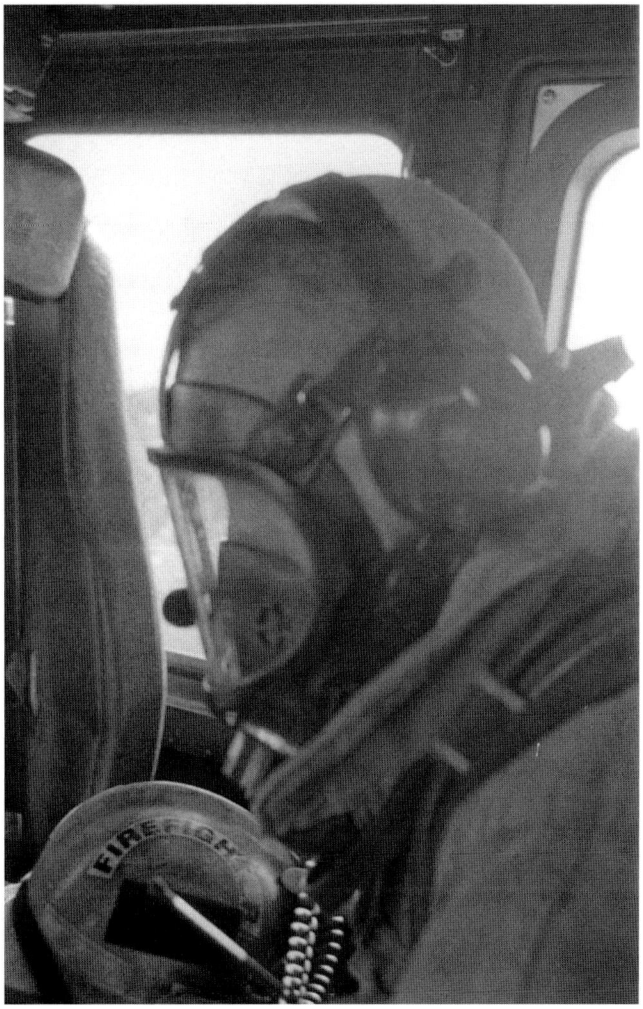

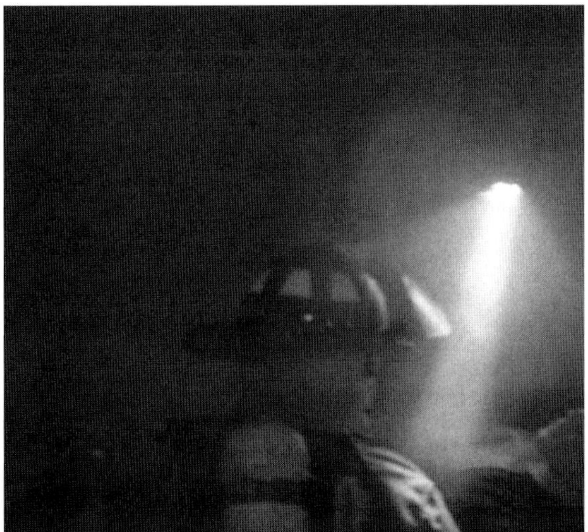

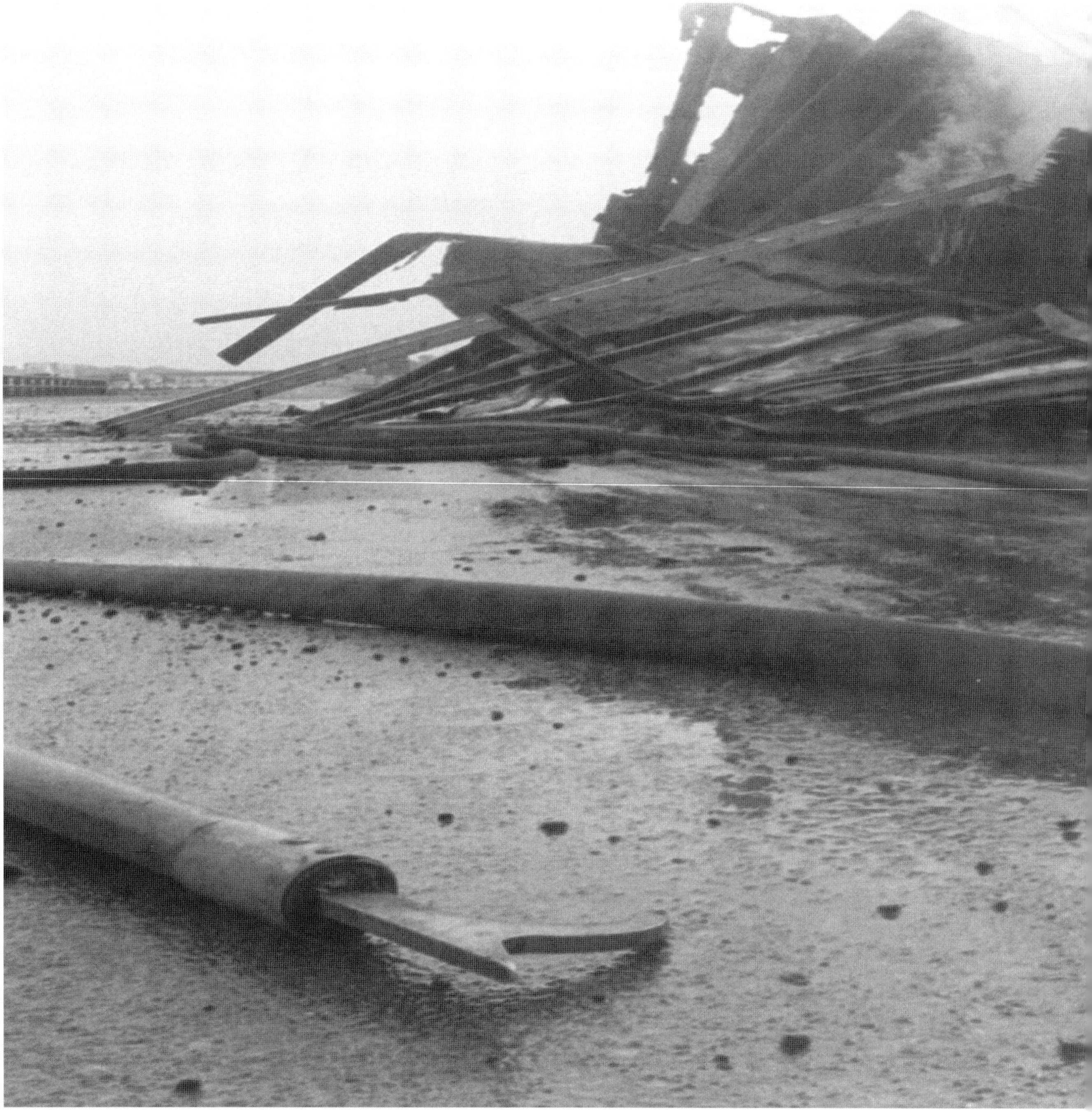

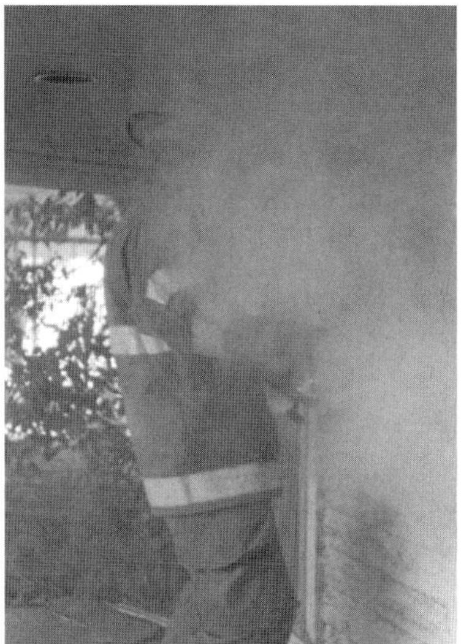

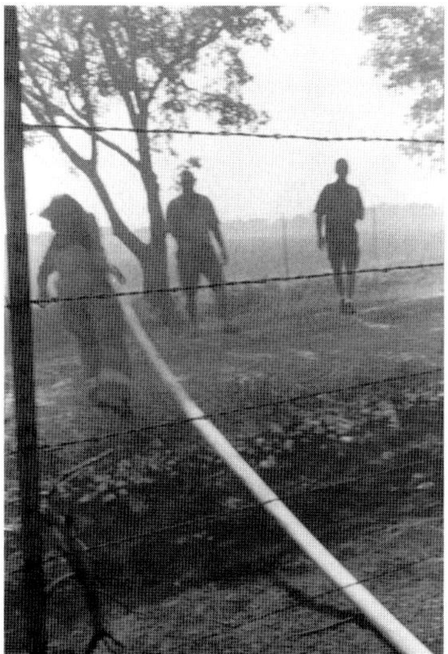

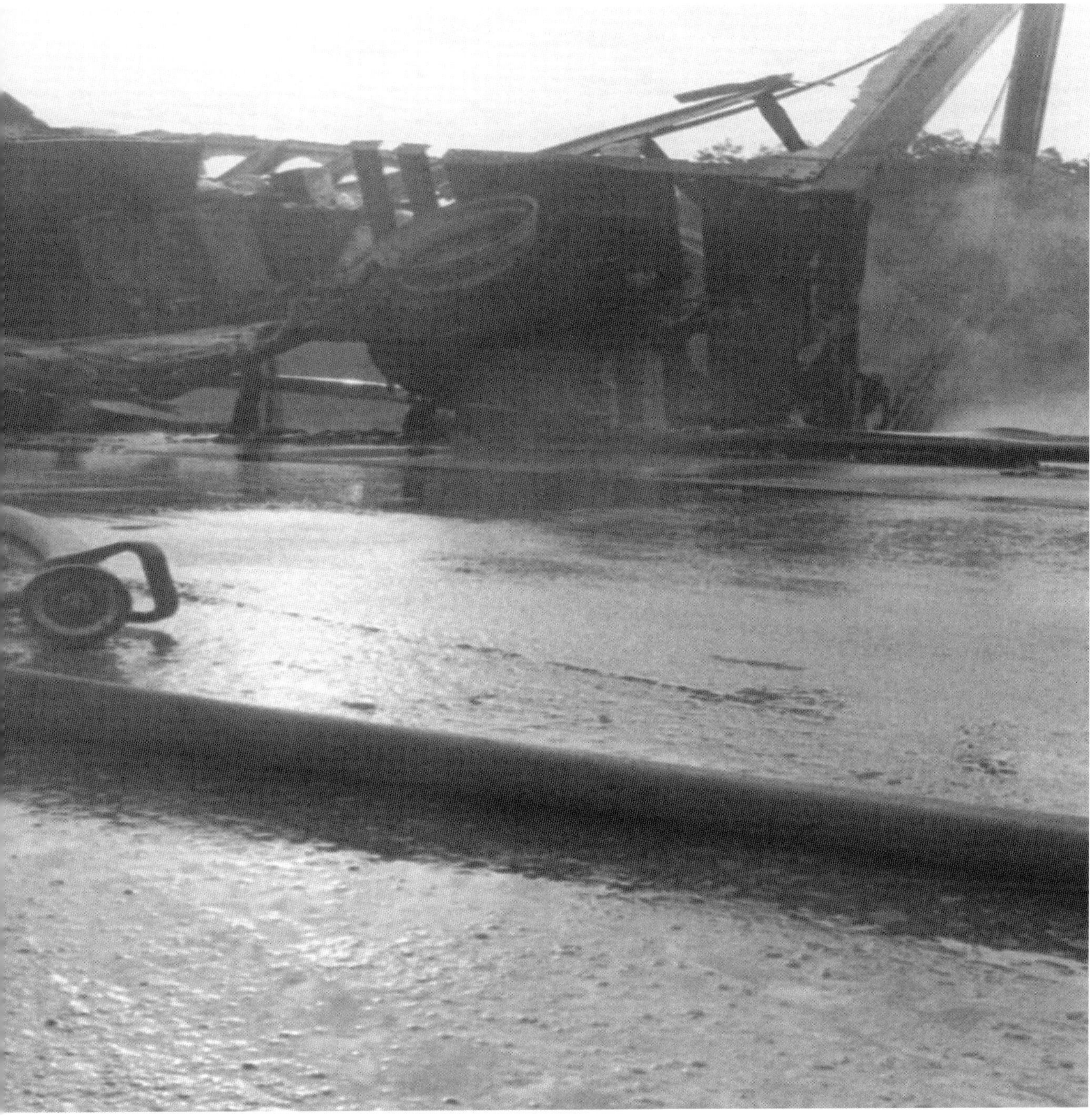

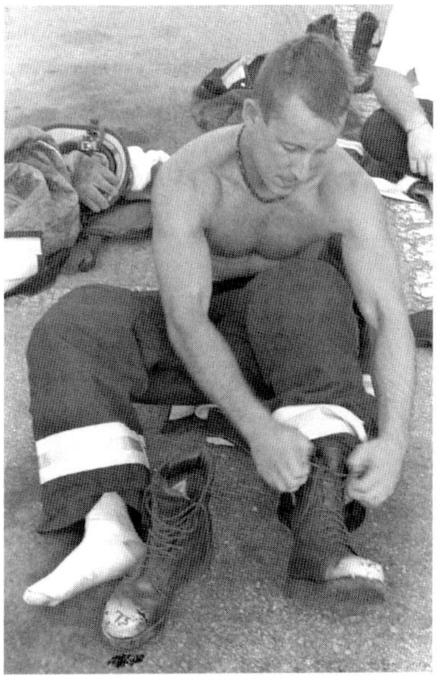

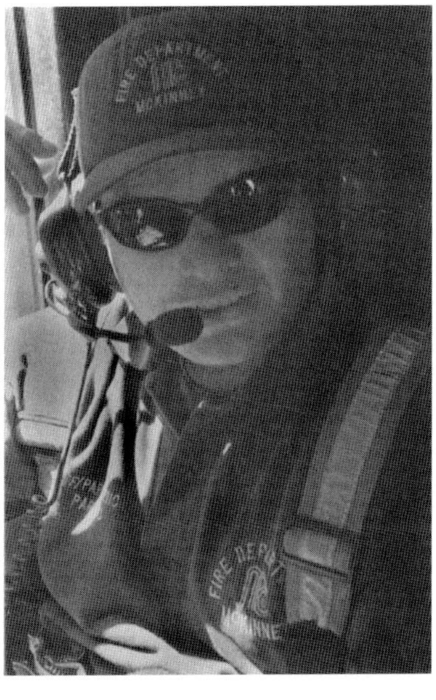

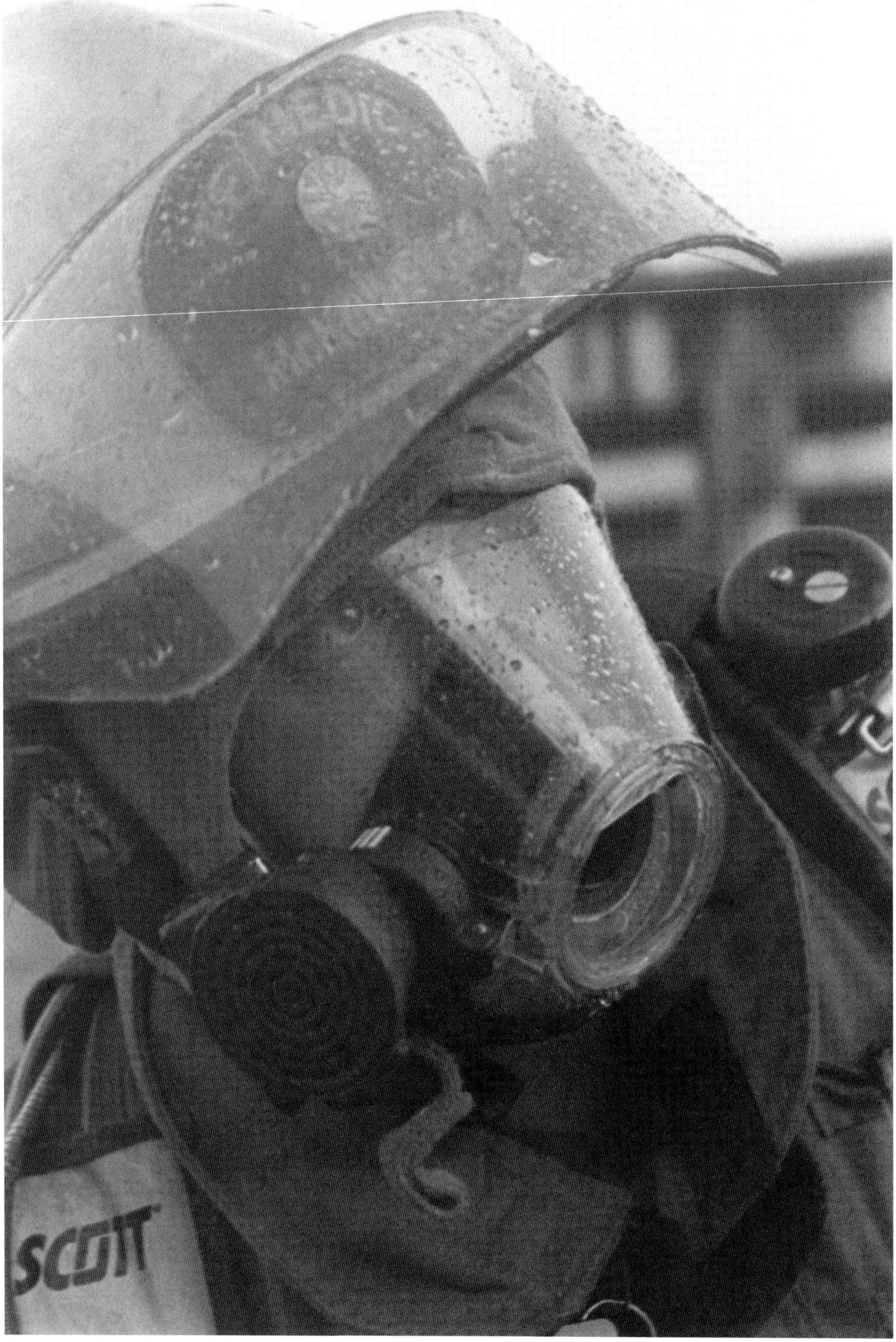
SCOTT

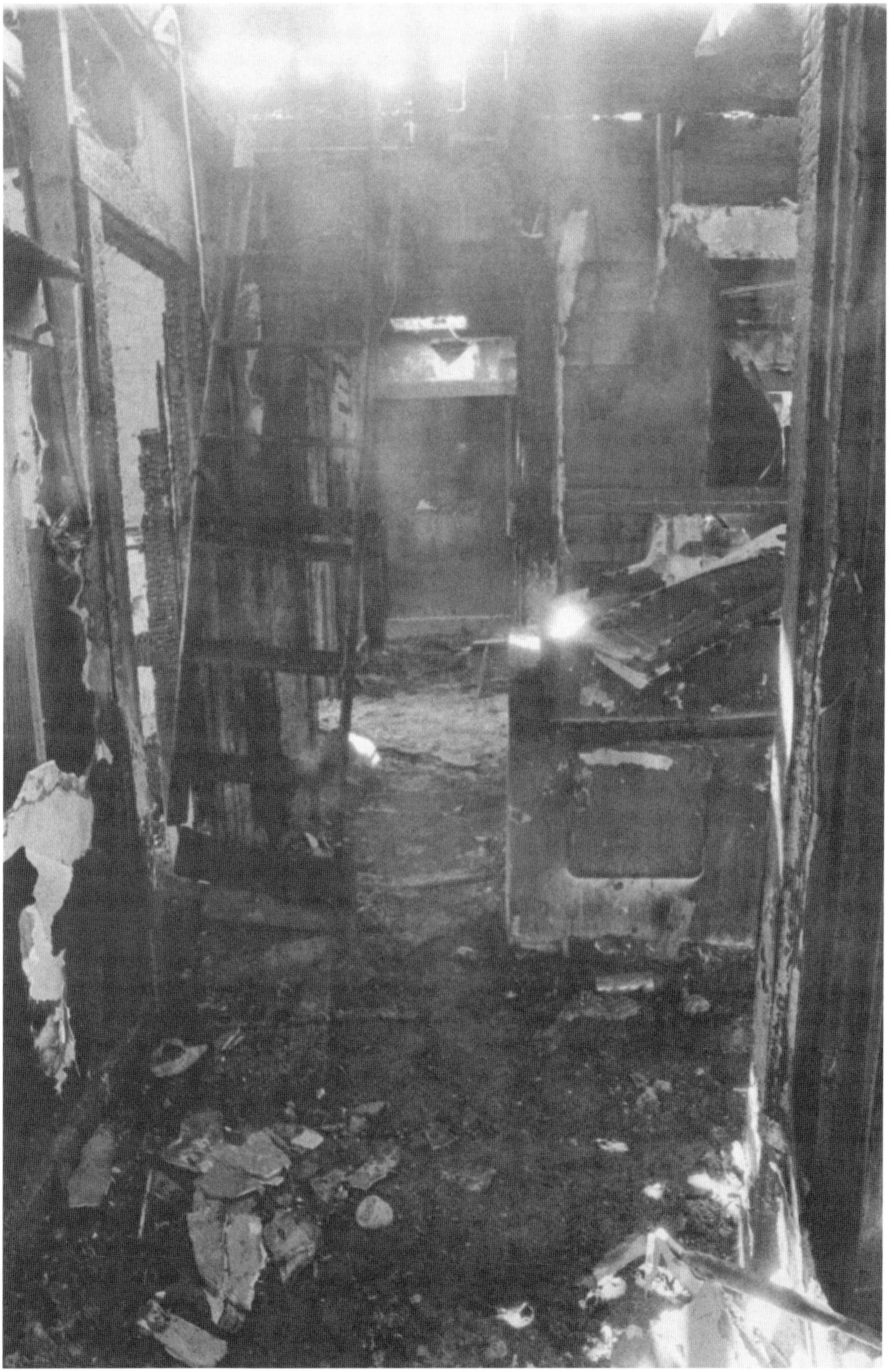

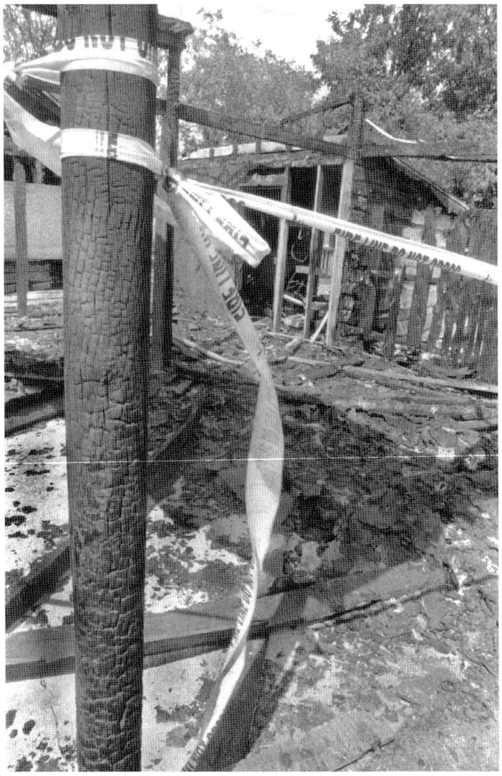

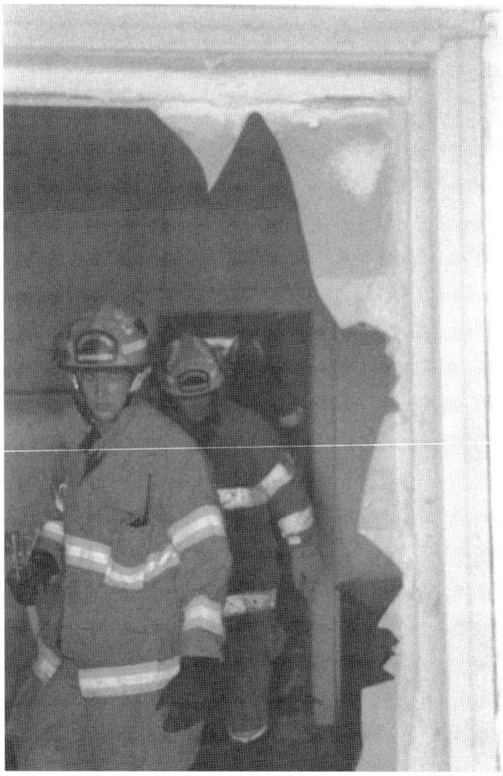

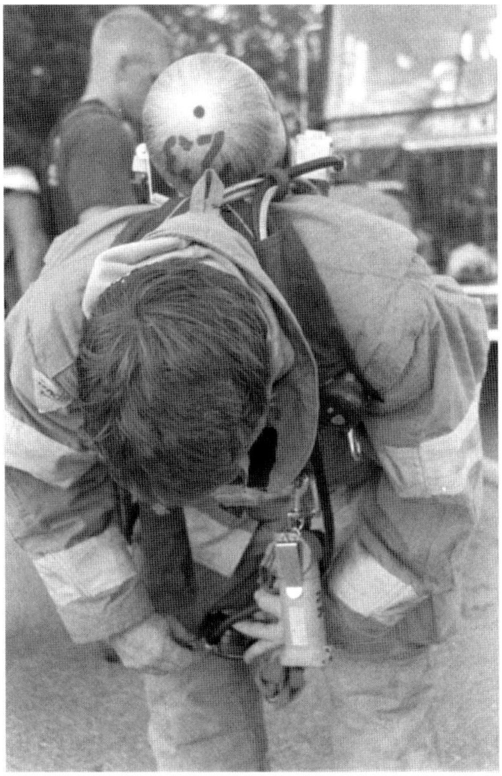

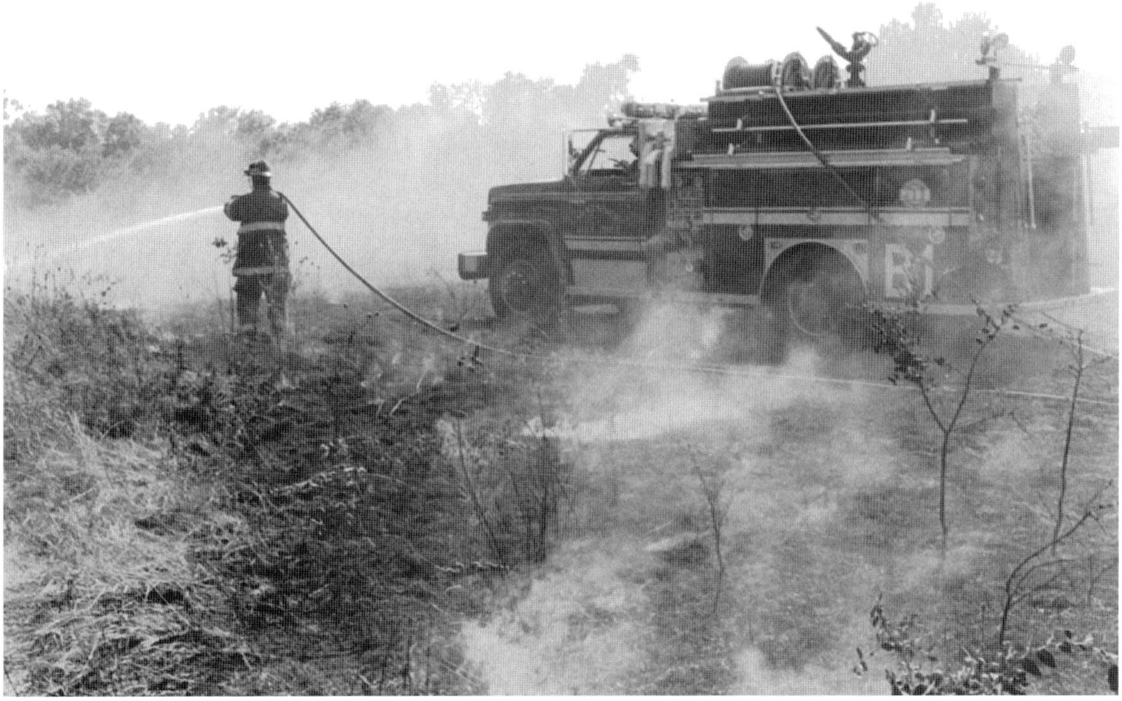
B1

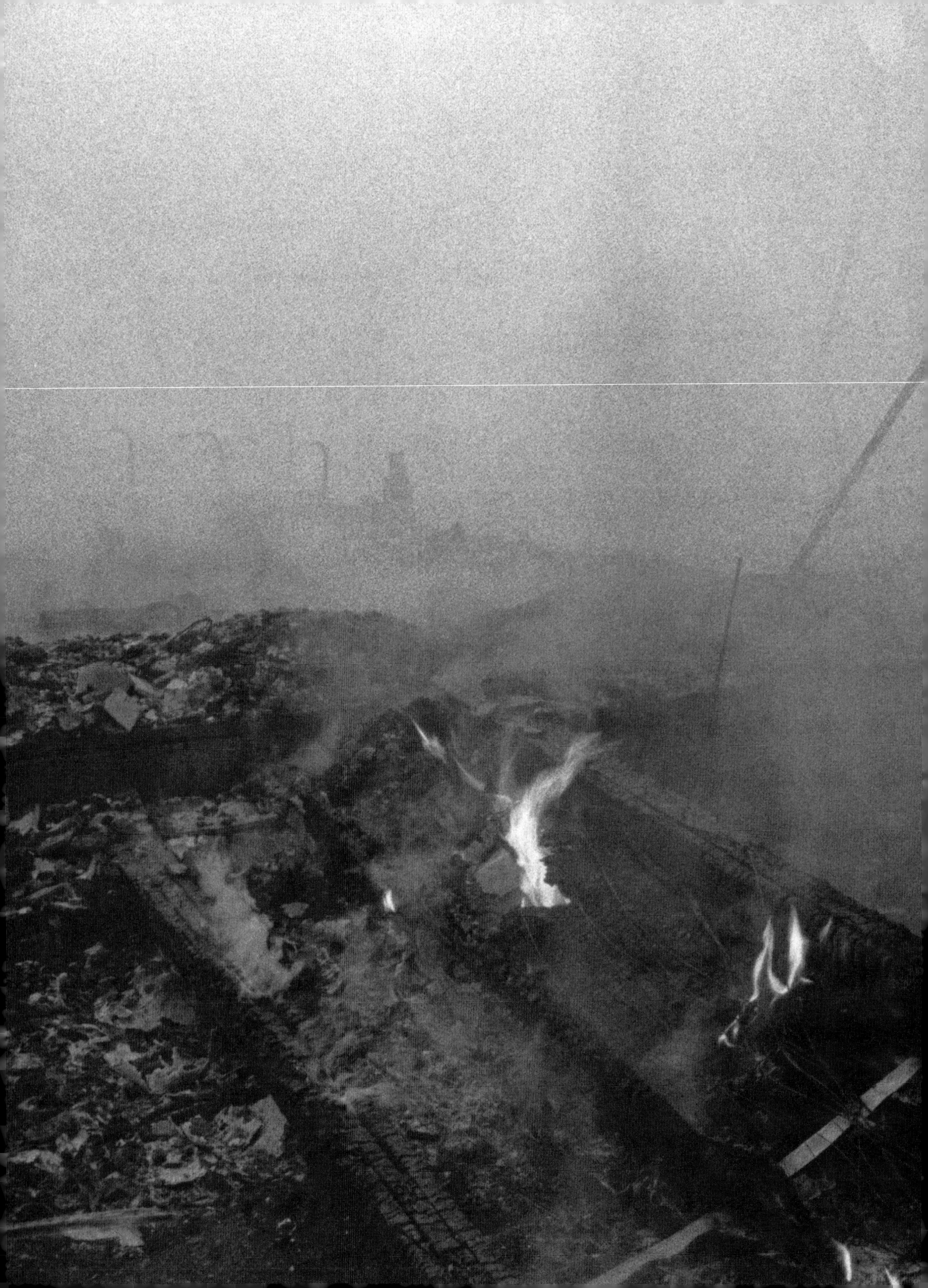

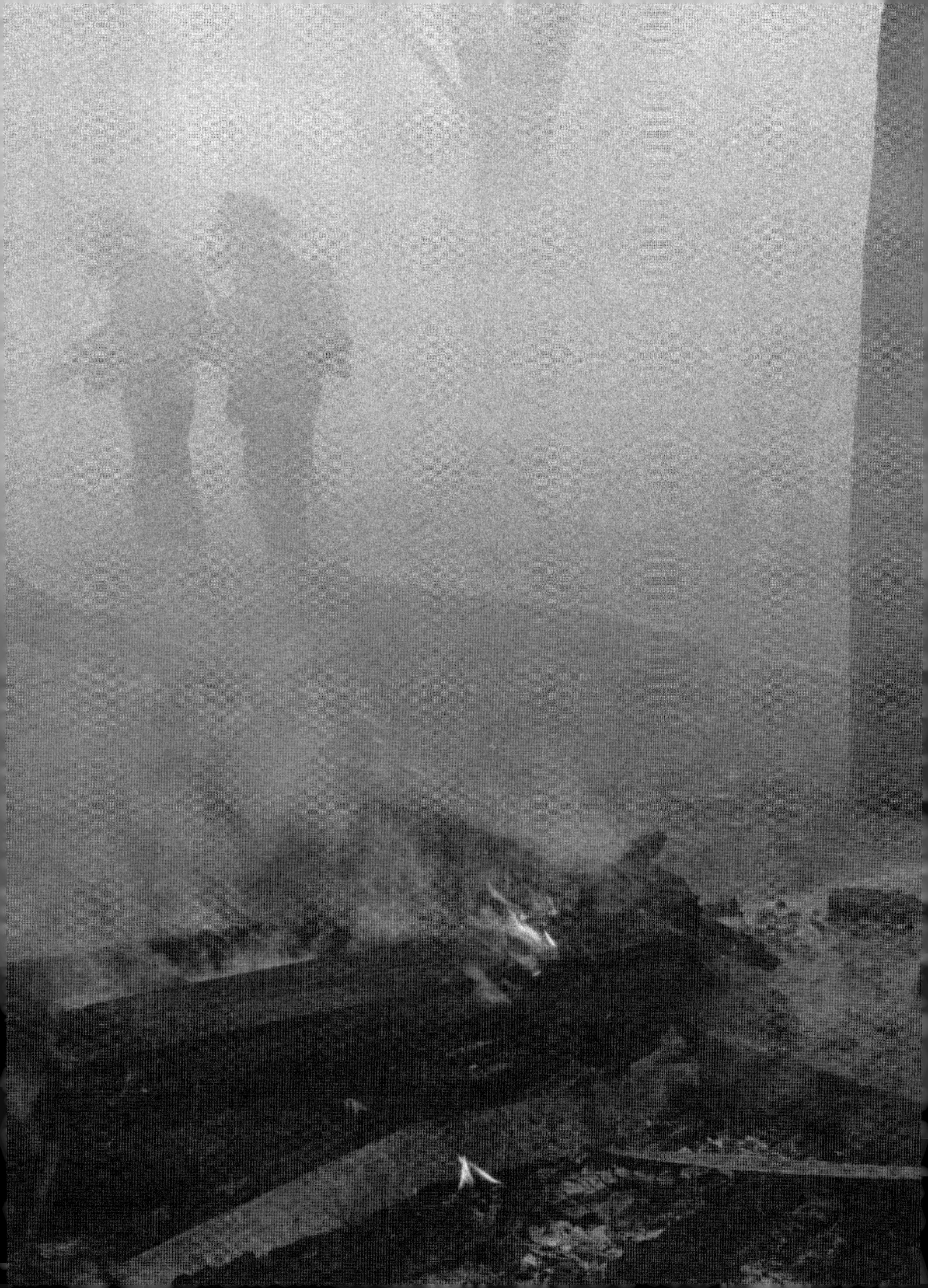

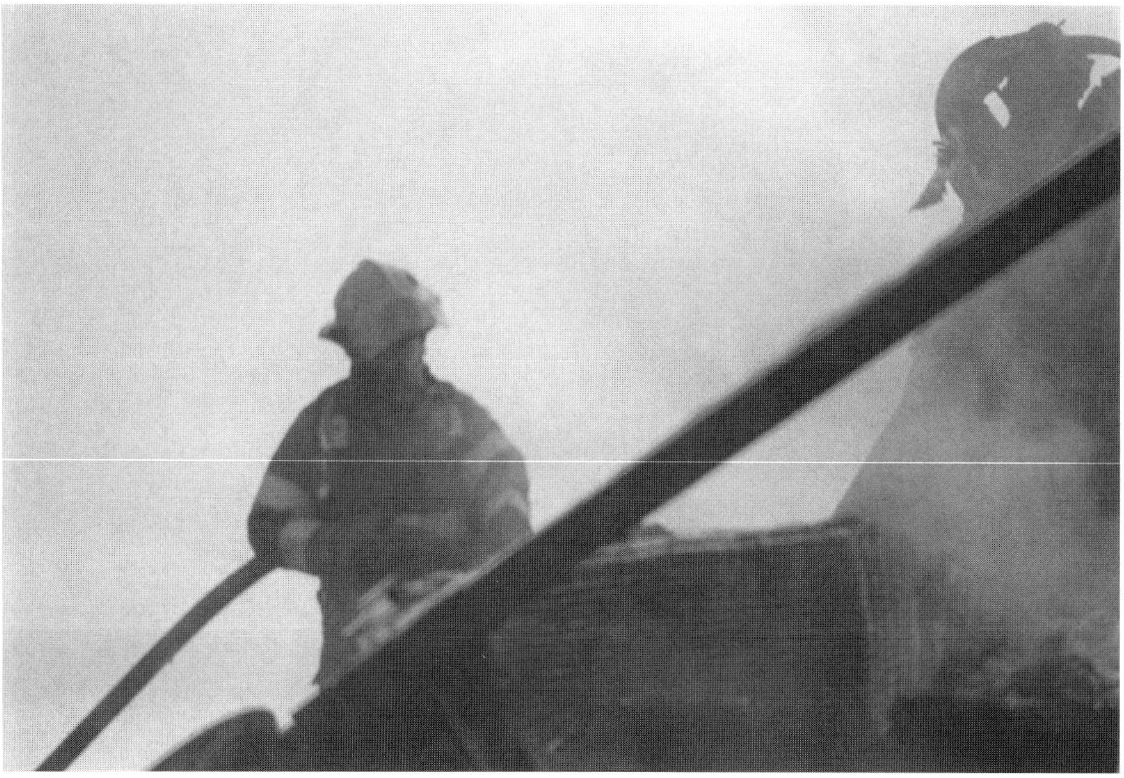

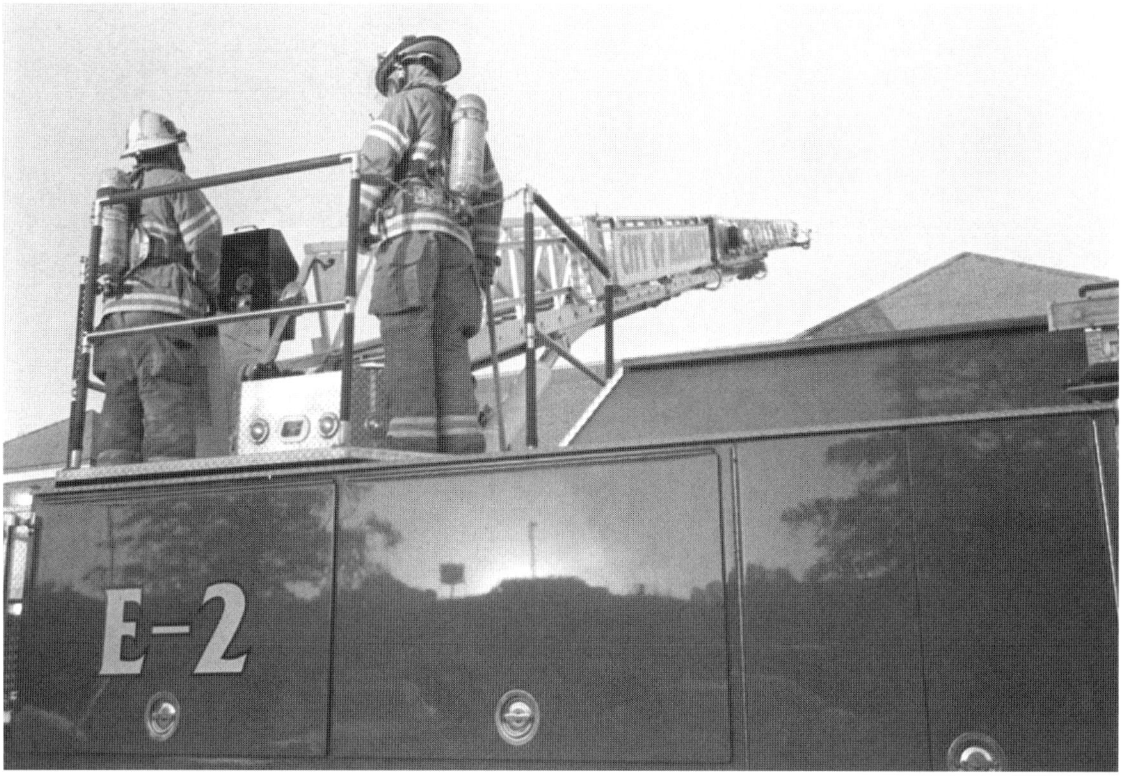
E-2

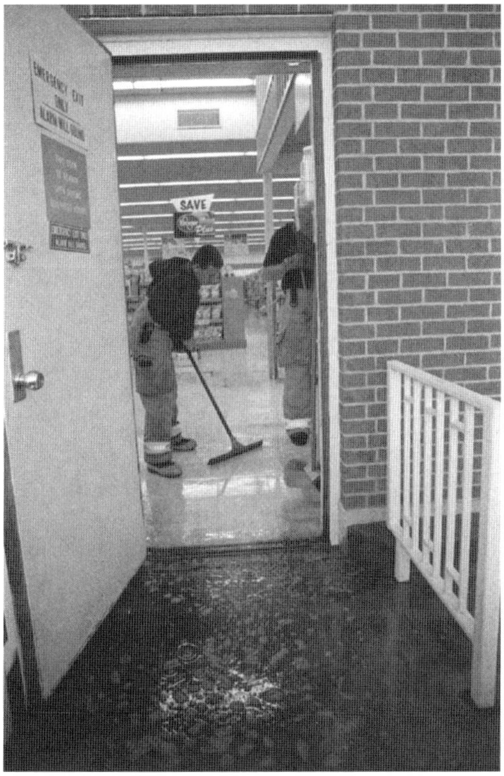
EMERGENCY EXIT
ONLY
ALARM WILL SOUND
SAVE

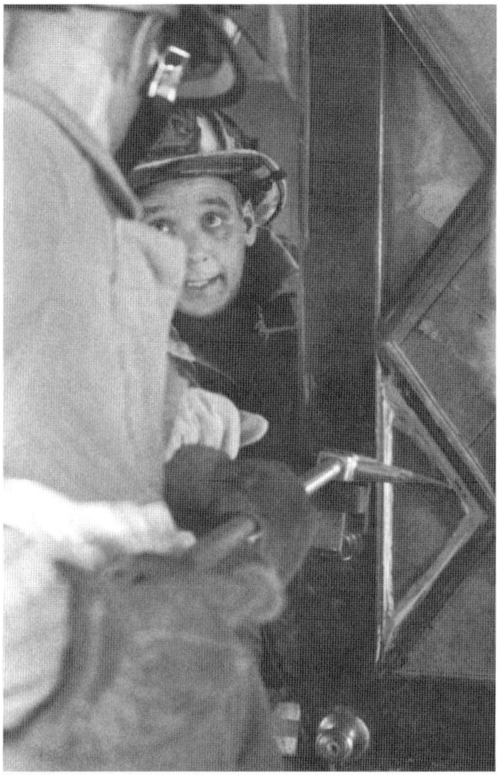

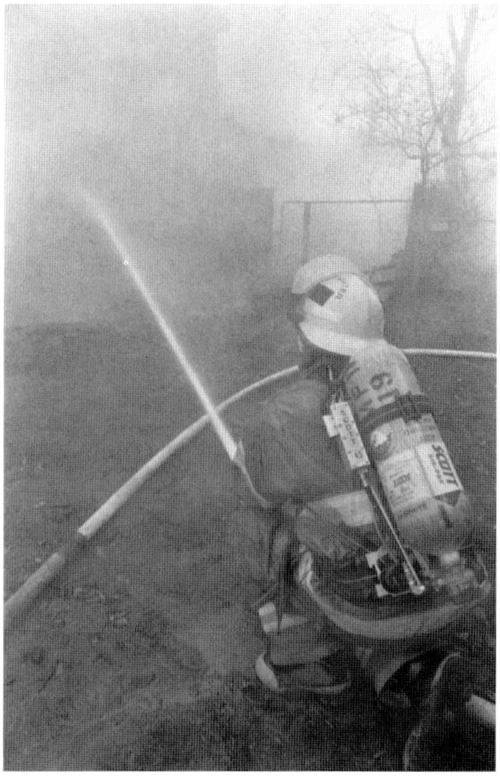

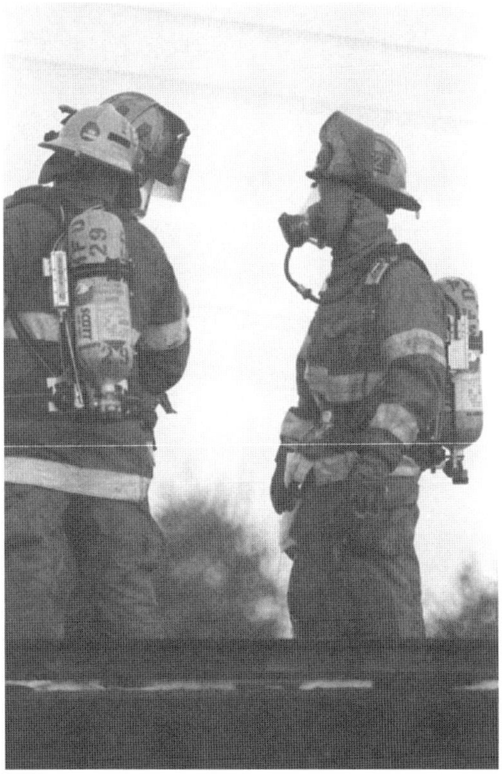

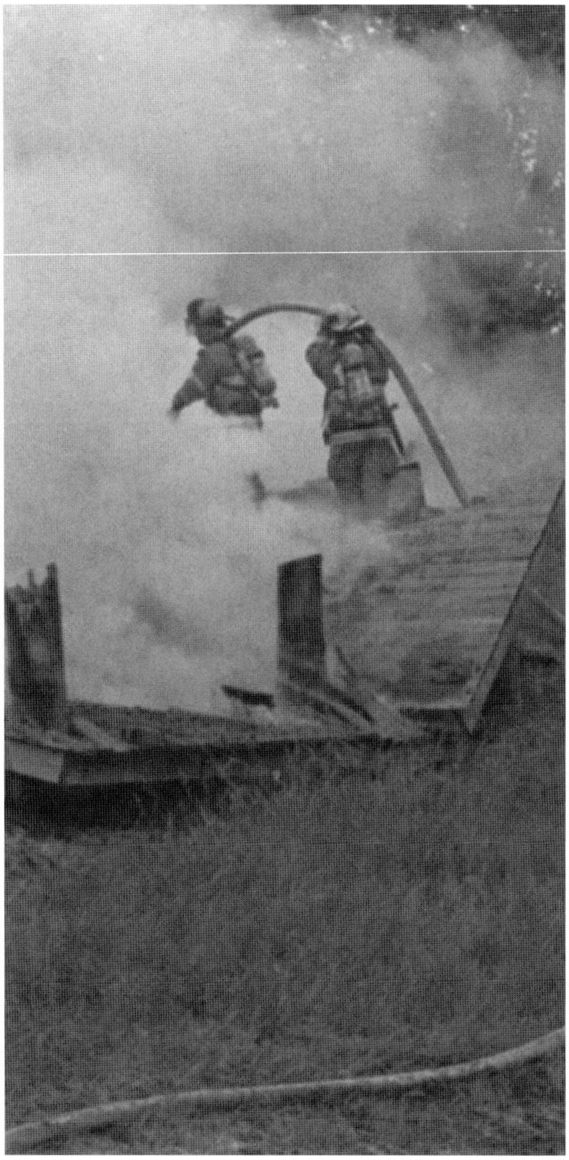

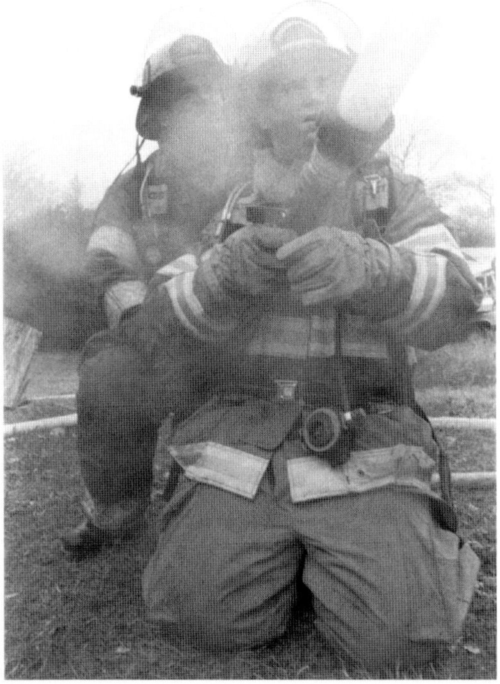

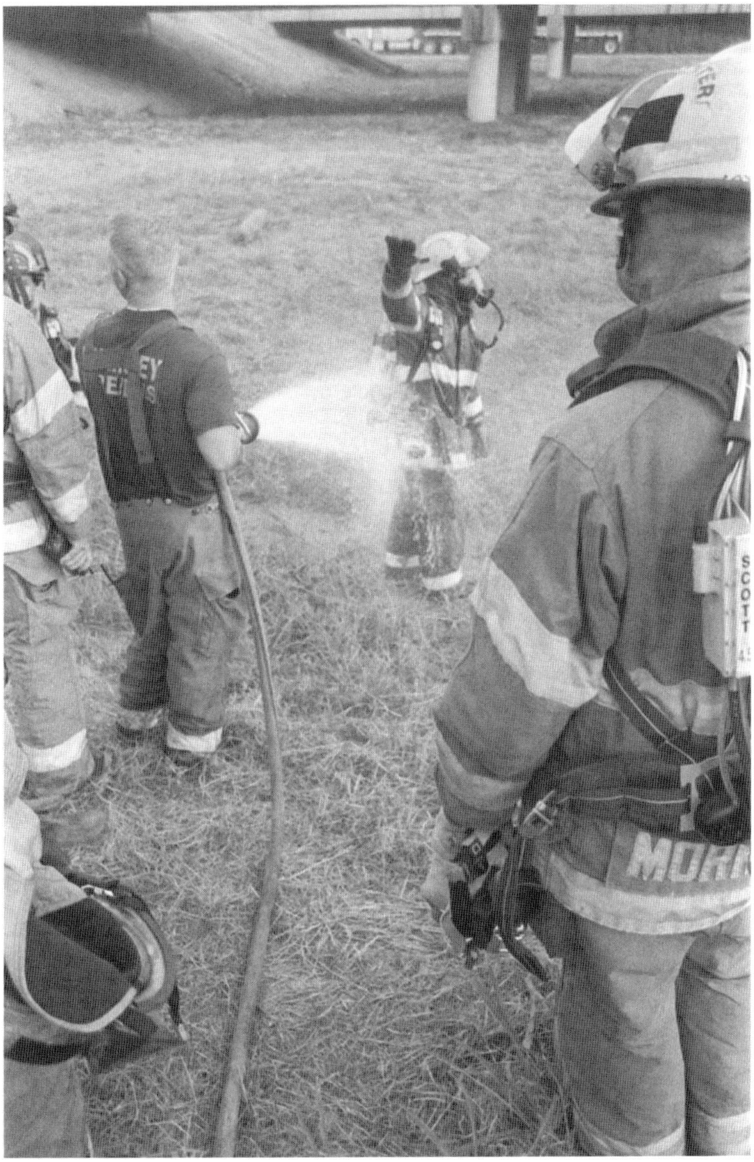
SCOTT
MORR

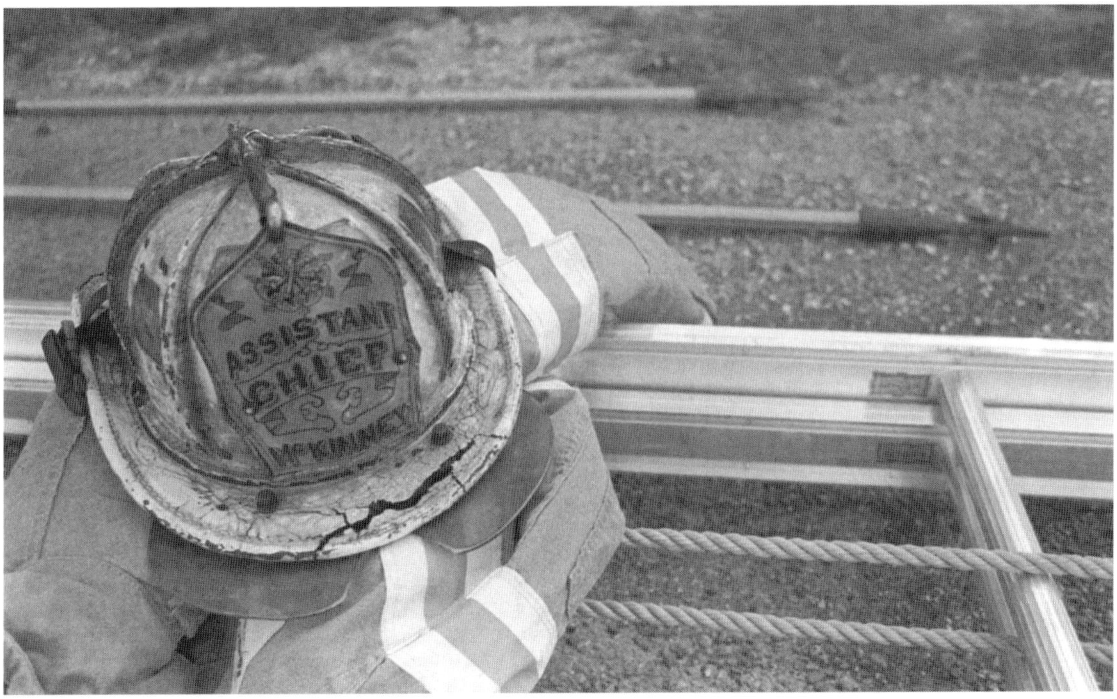
ASSISTANT
CHIEF
McKINNEY

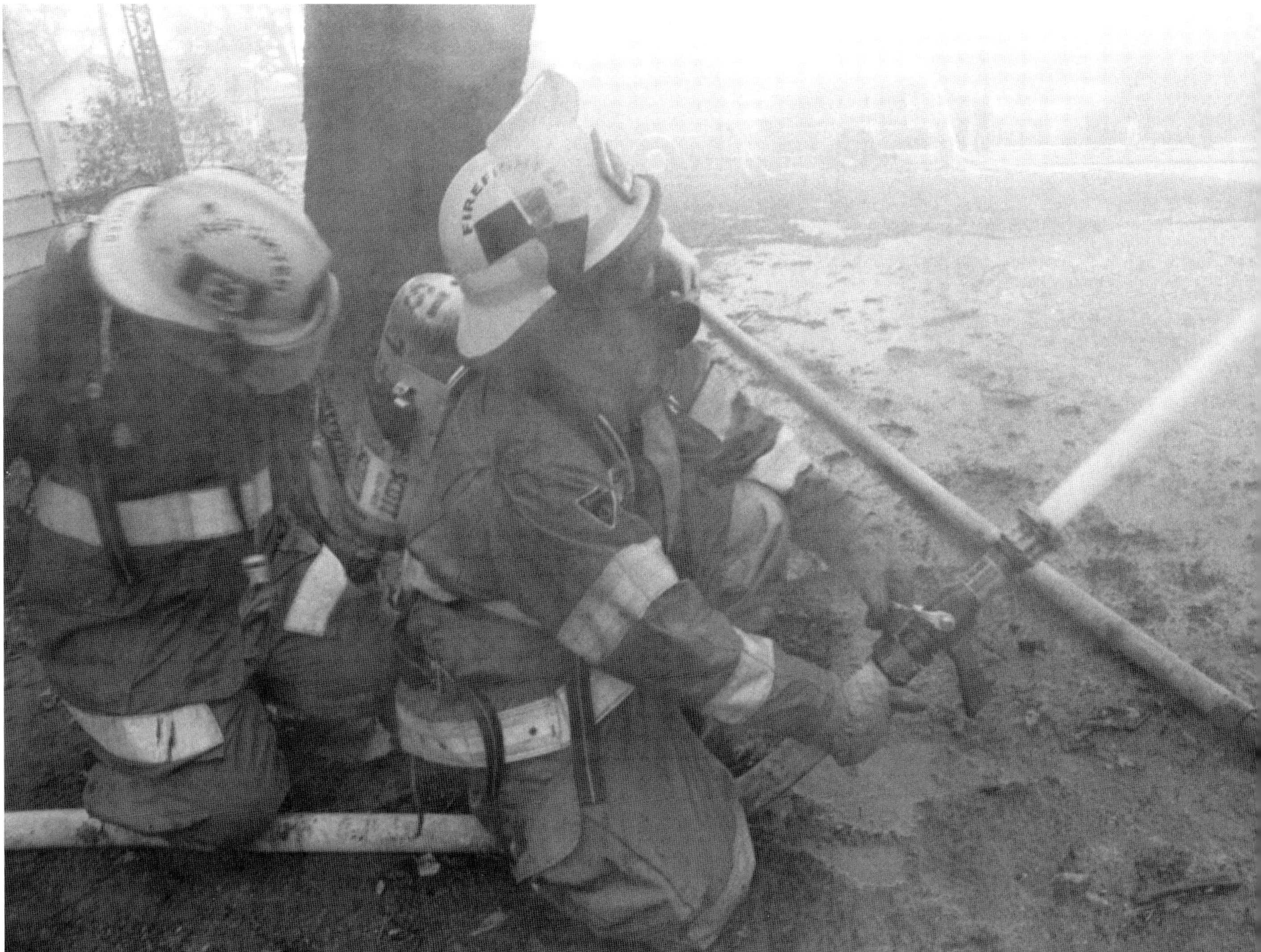

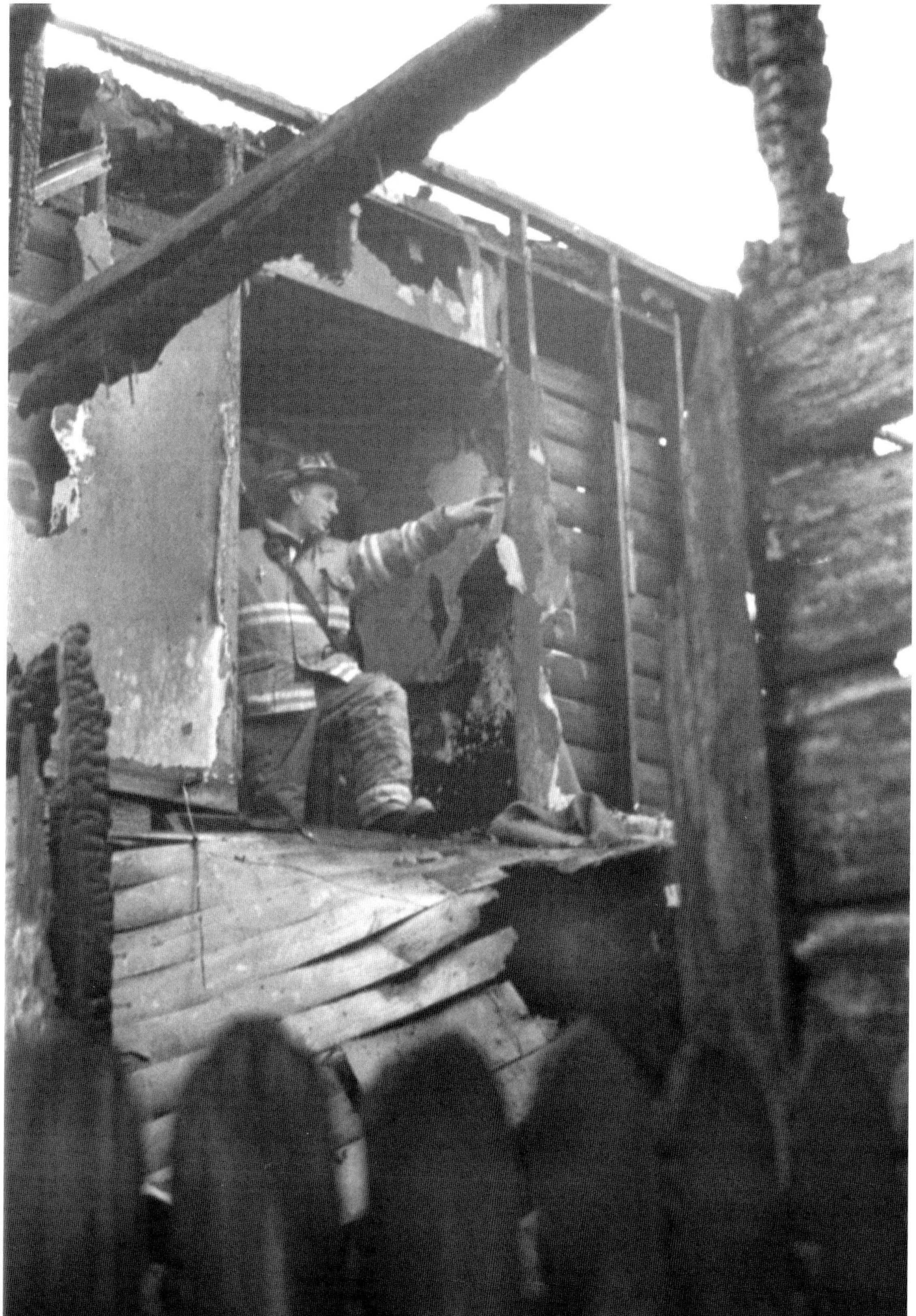

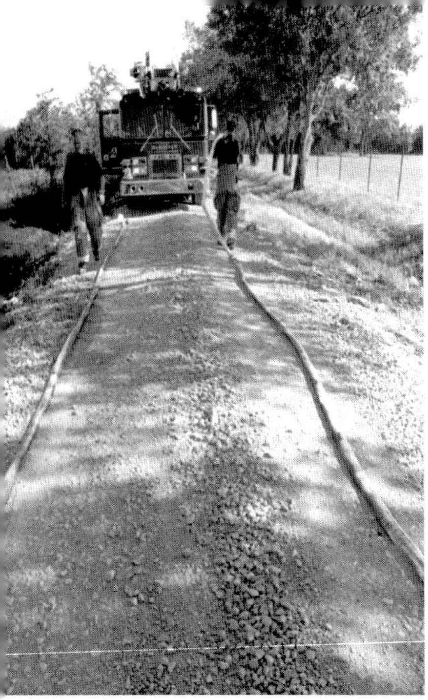

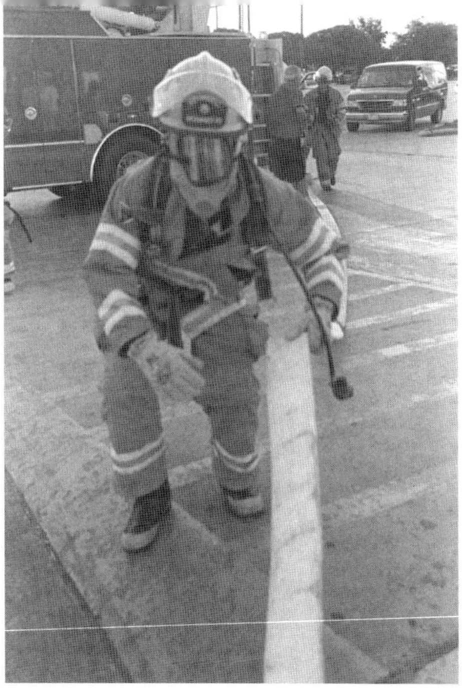

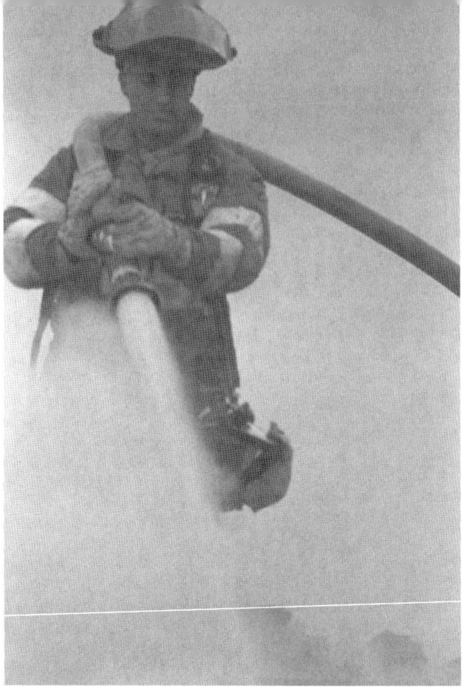

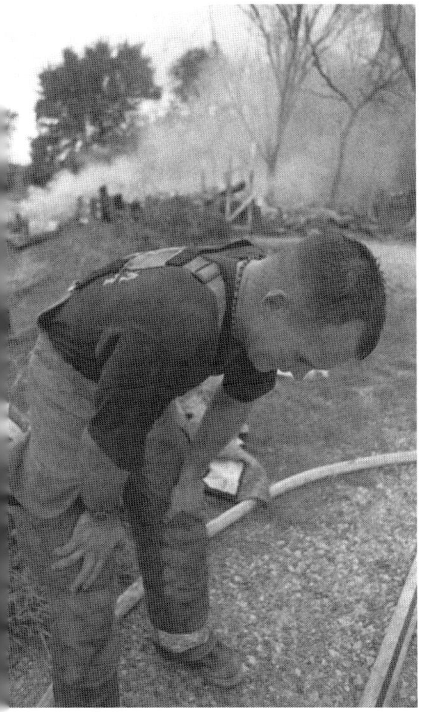

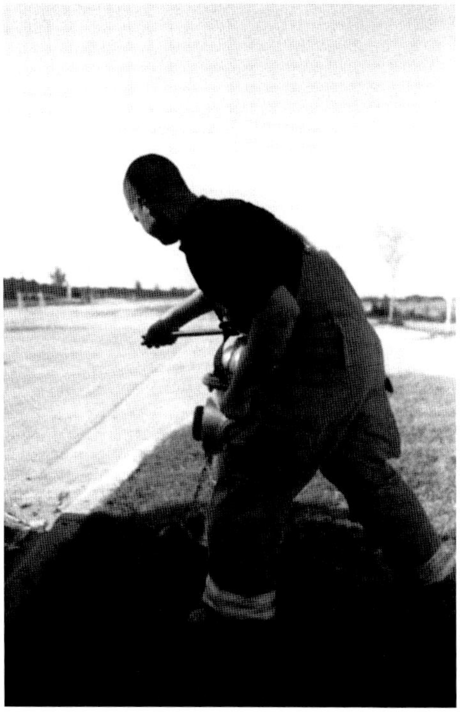

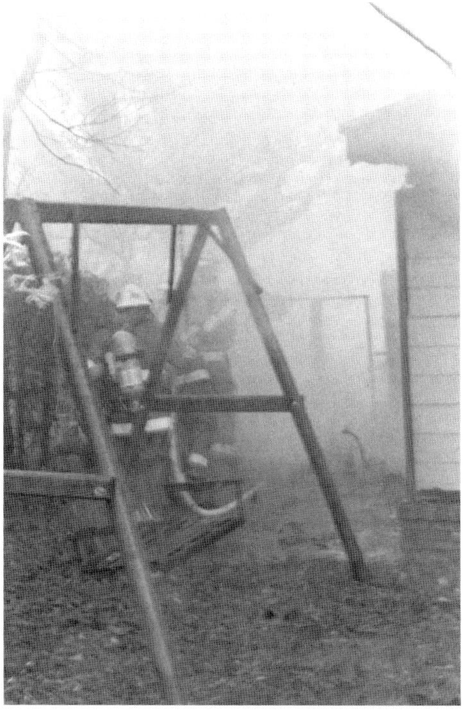

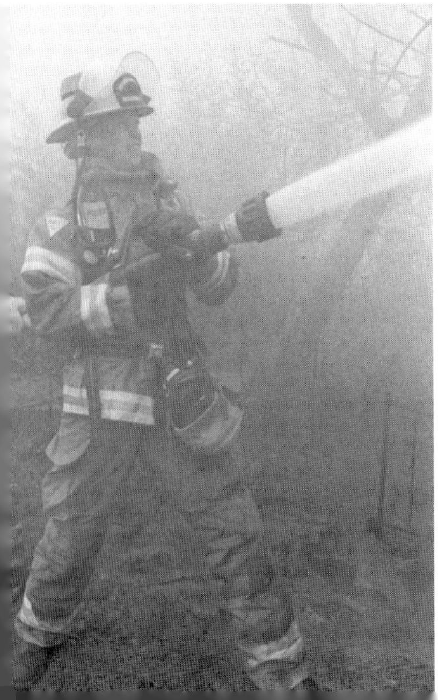

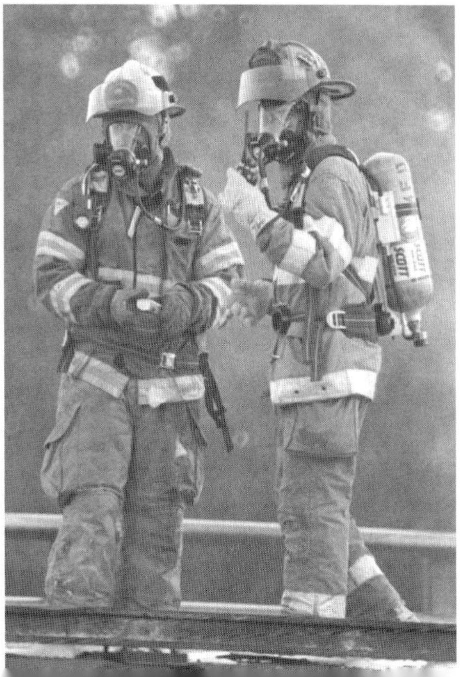
SCOTT

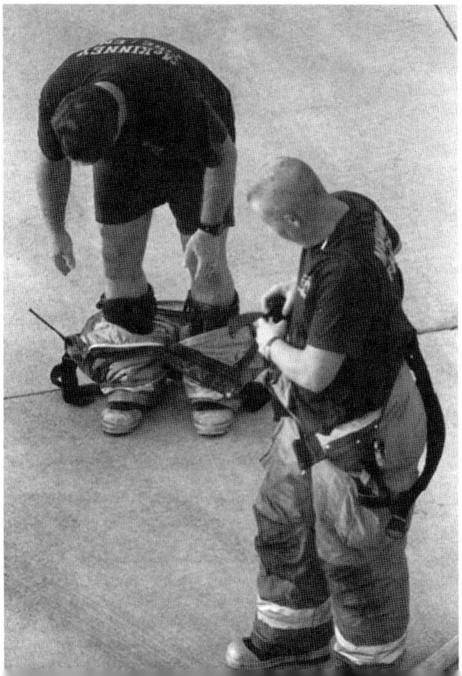

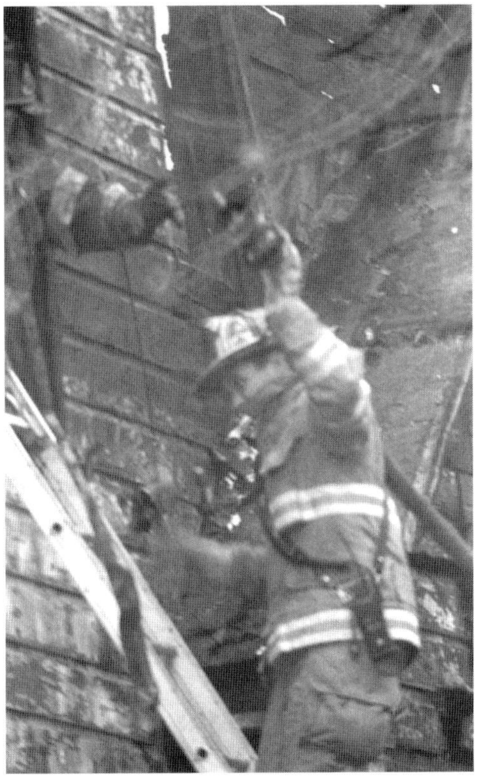

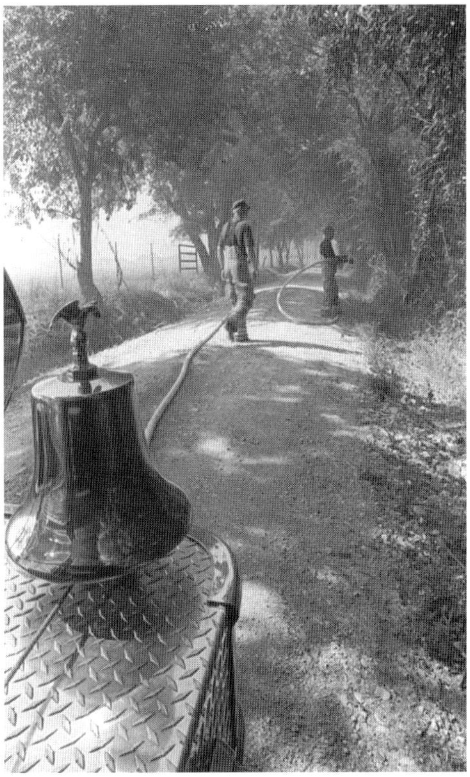

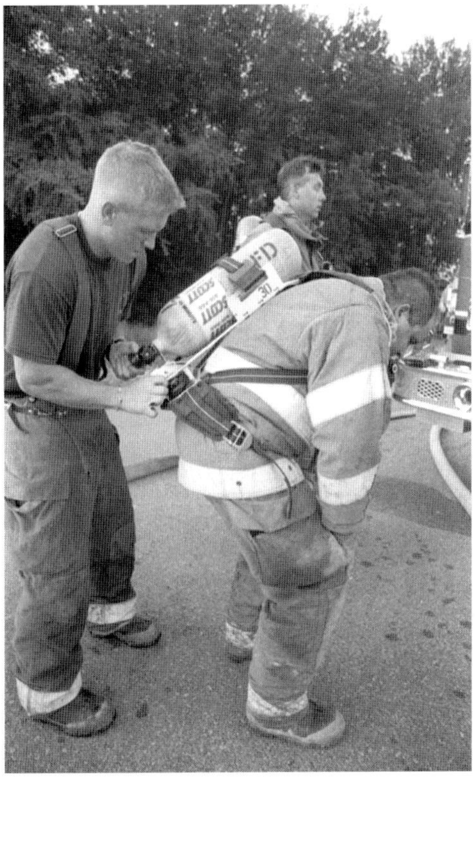
SCOTT
30

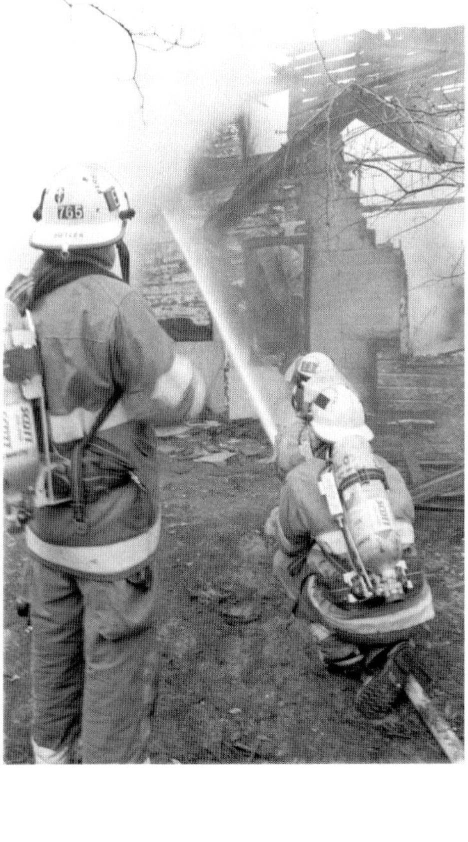
765

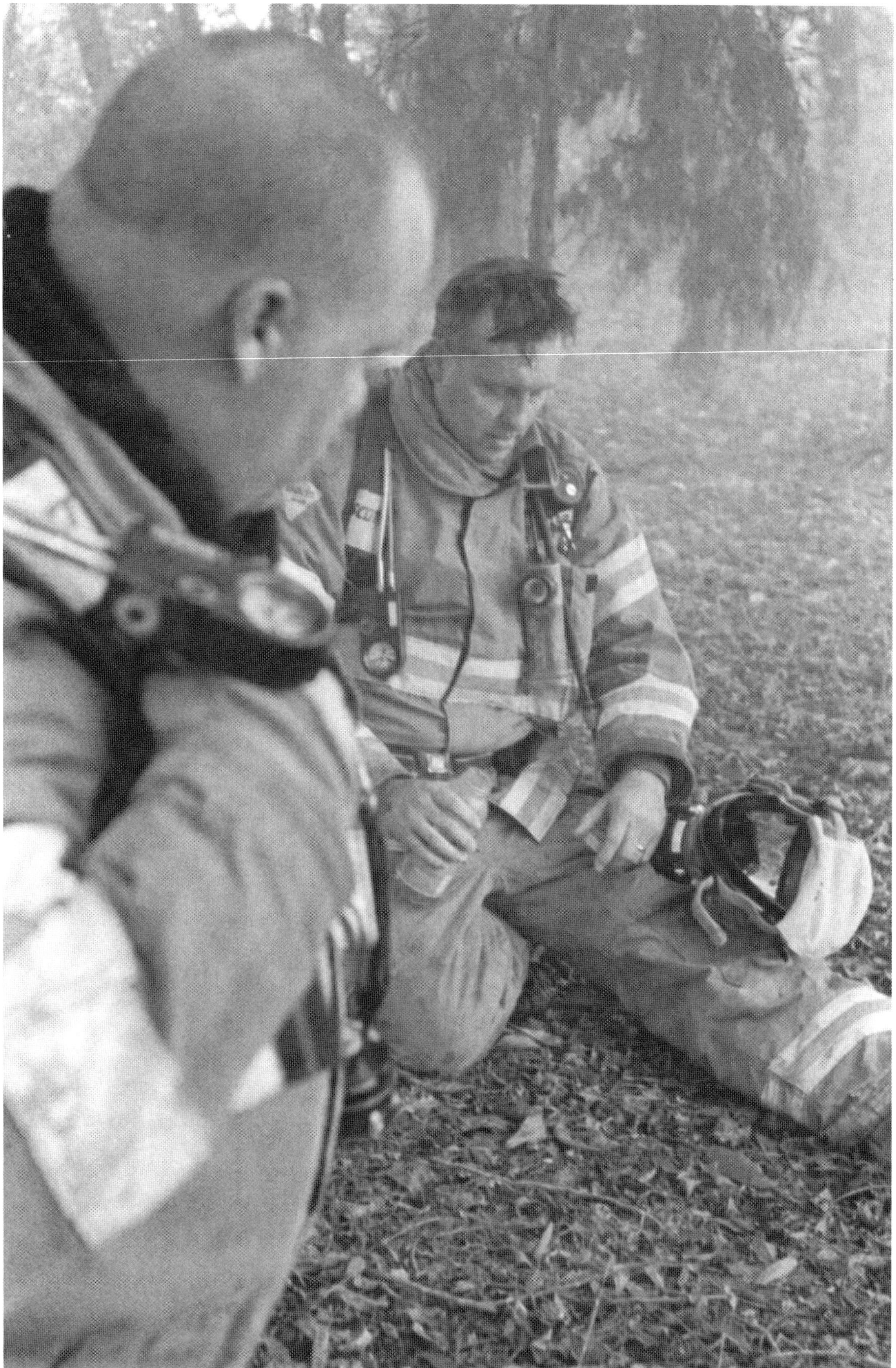

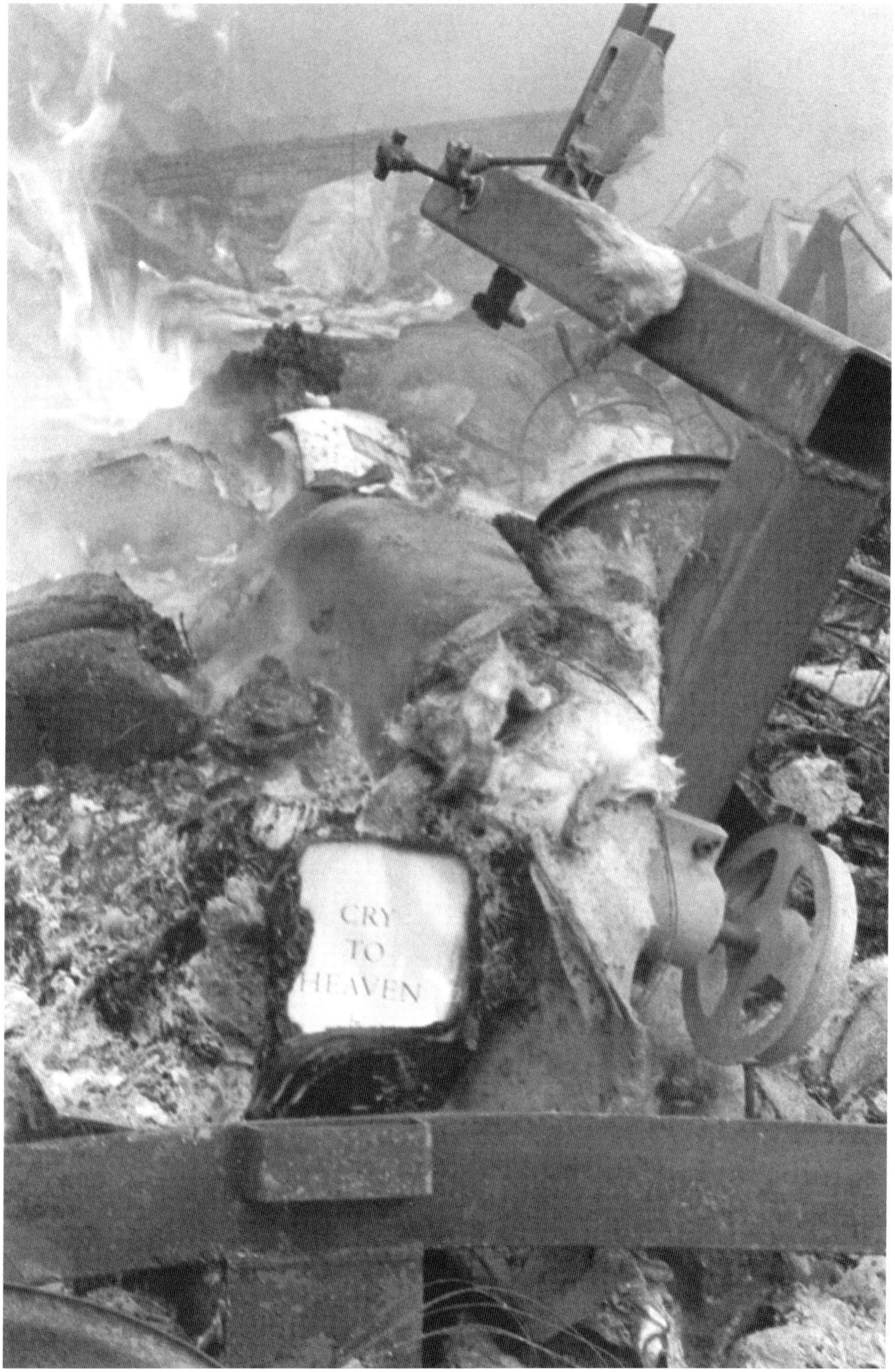
CRY
TO
HEAVEN

# station

Call it station, call it office, call it house, home and haven for the men and women of your local fire department. They do what we do in our places... and more. It is their 24 hour scene for school, and work, and life.

"Have we tested all the equipment?" "Who's cooking?" "Whatcha want for breakfast? How 'bout lunch? Dinner?" "What's the training schedule today?" "Is there Blue Bell in the fridge?" "What time does the game start on TV tonight?" "Clean the head!" "Hey Don, your wife's on line one." And above all this, is the call out alarm... ***"Engine two, Med one***"... life stops in the house and sirens wail into the distance toward a critical destination.

Between fire and medical runs, the firestation or 'house' is a Firefighters safe harbor to wash, sleep, train, relax, cook, worry, eat, study, talk, clean, smile, poke fun, tell jokes, laugh, think, play, and do all the things that occupy each of us on our journey through each day and night. Like most homes, firestations have beds and bedrooms, showers and stalls, kitchens, TV and dining rooms, study and office areas, storage bins, washer/dryers, a big garage... you name it.

All the pleasures and heartaches we all experience with our families at our home, they do in theirs. Firefighters are a very special family that live in a very special house.

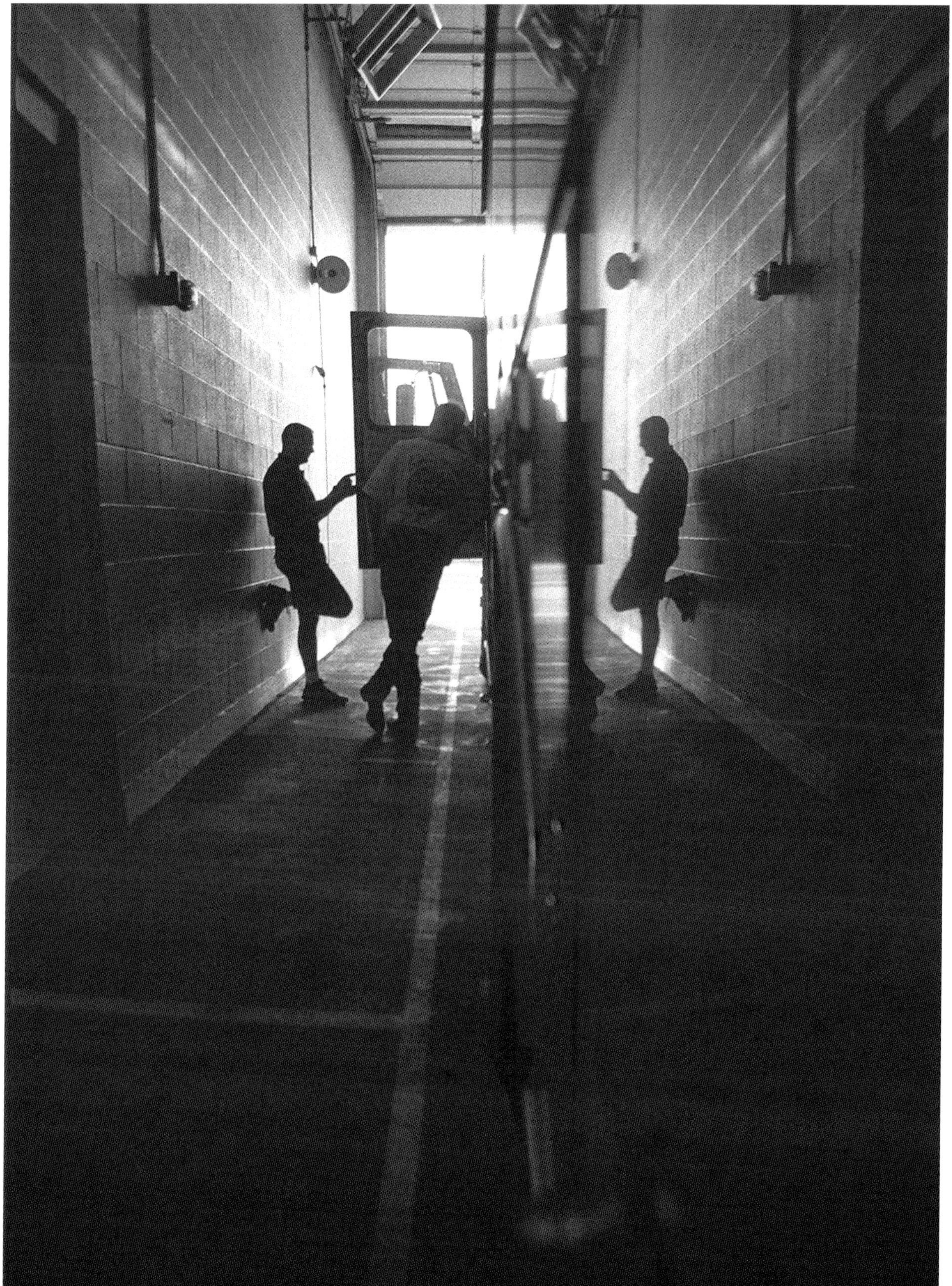

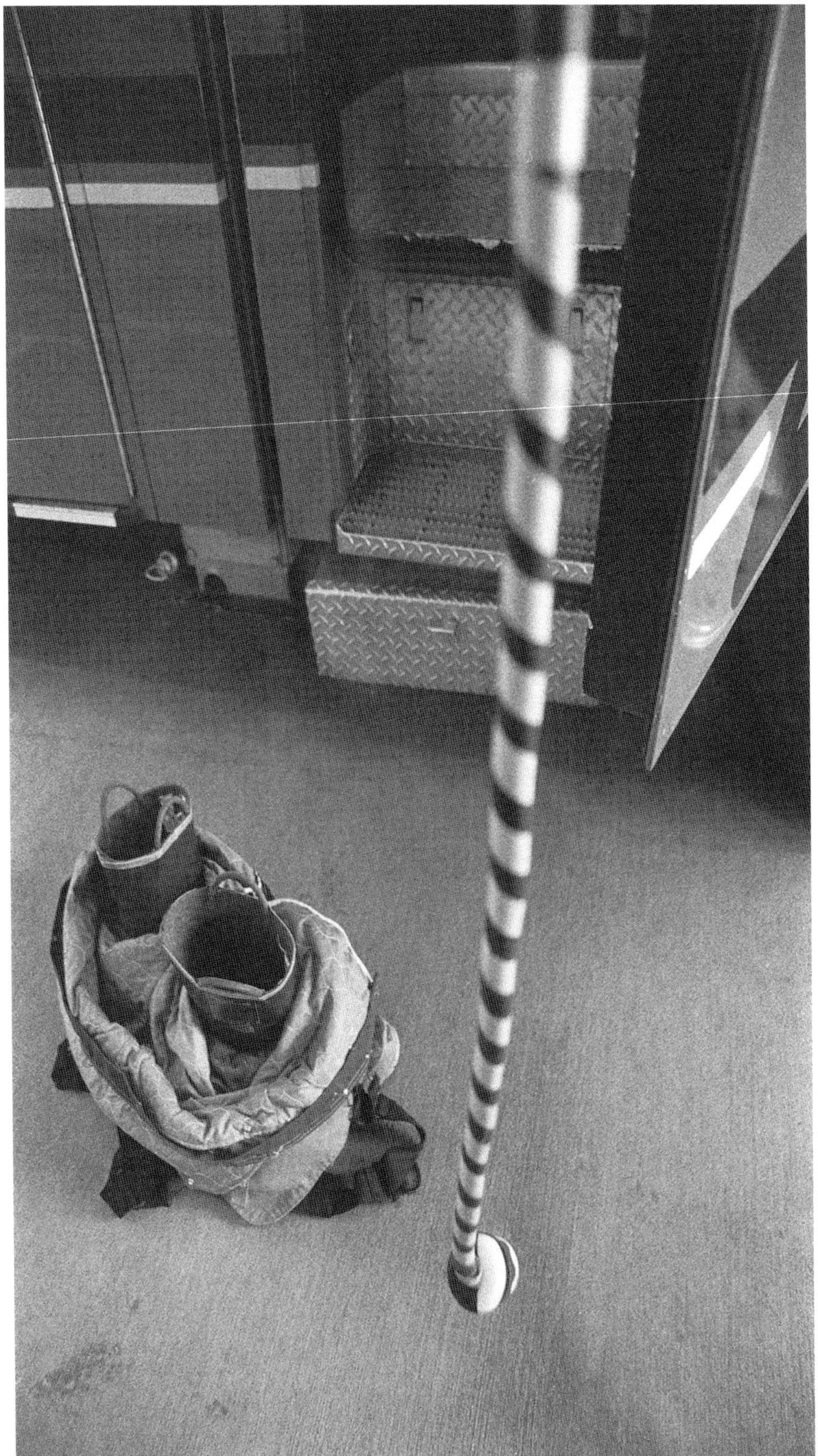

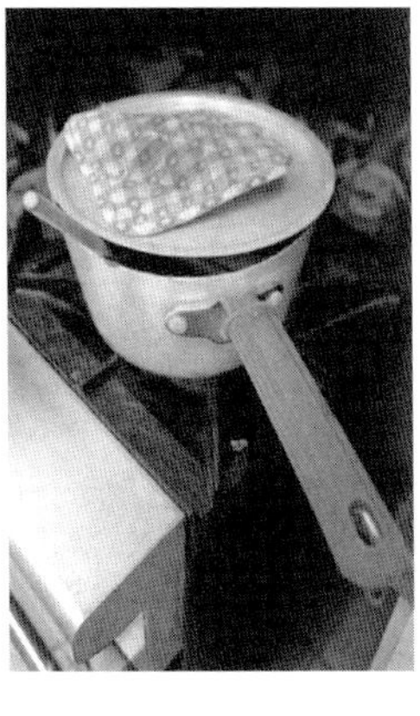

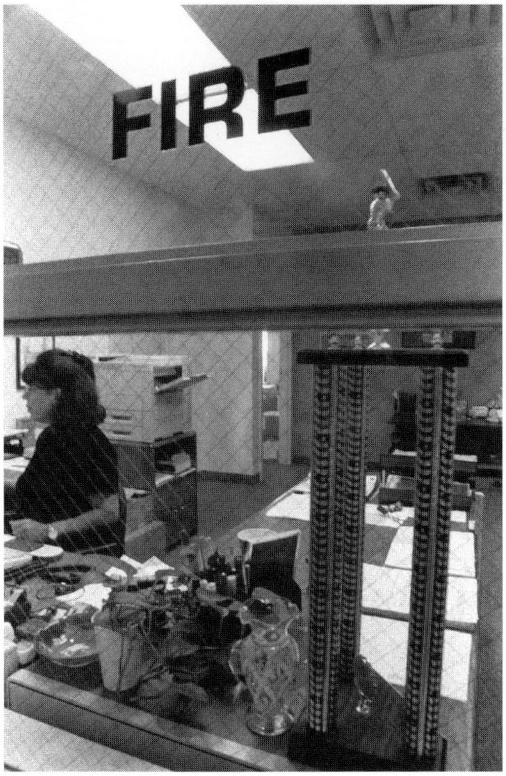
FIRE

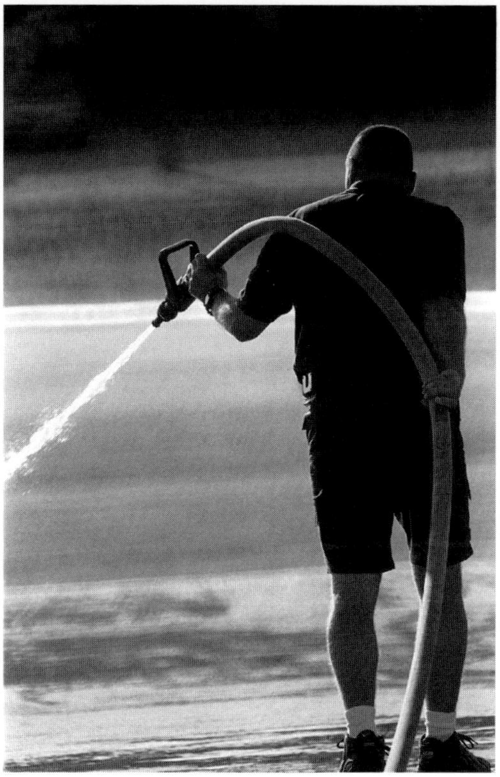

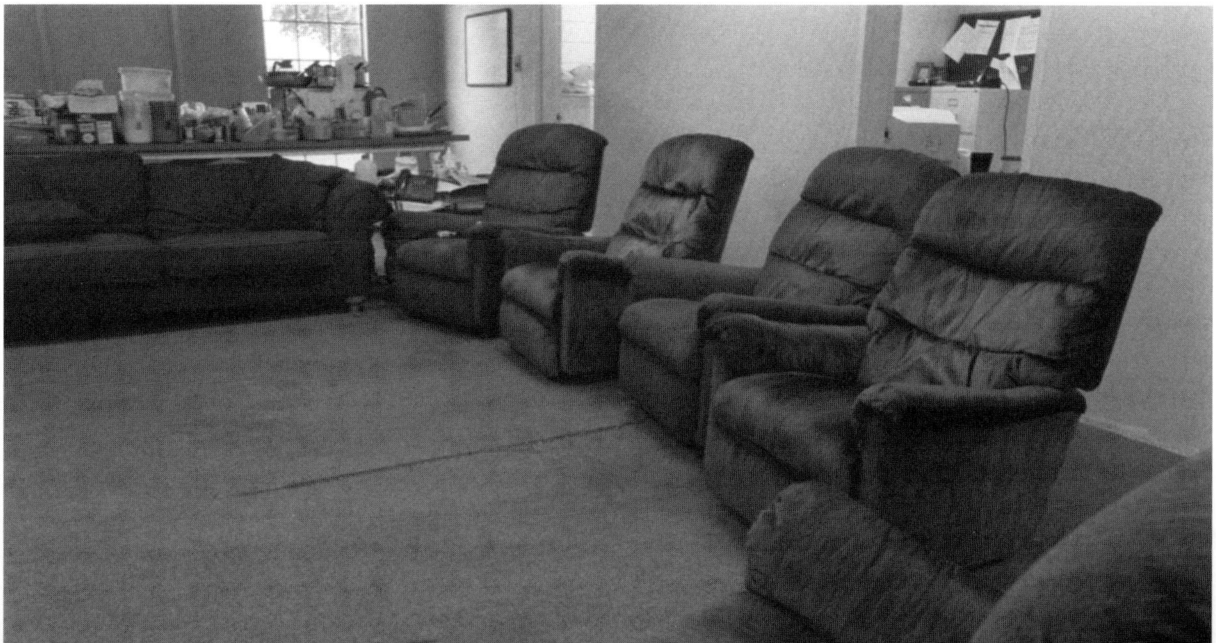

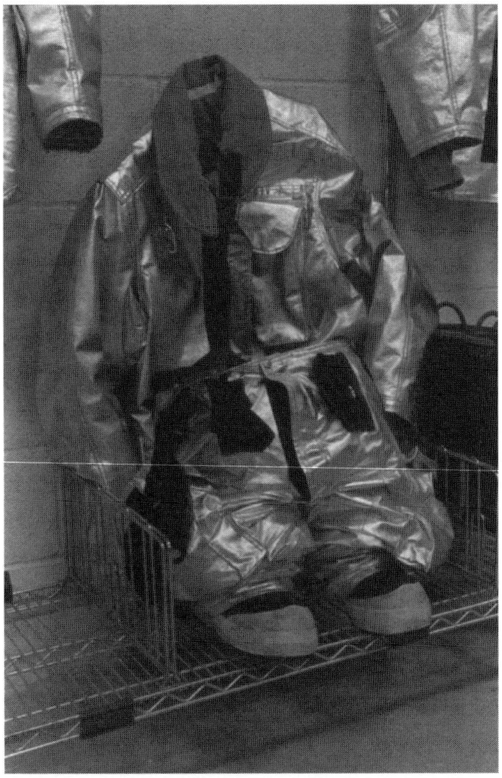

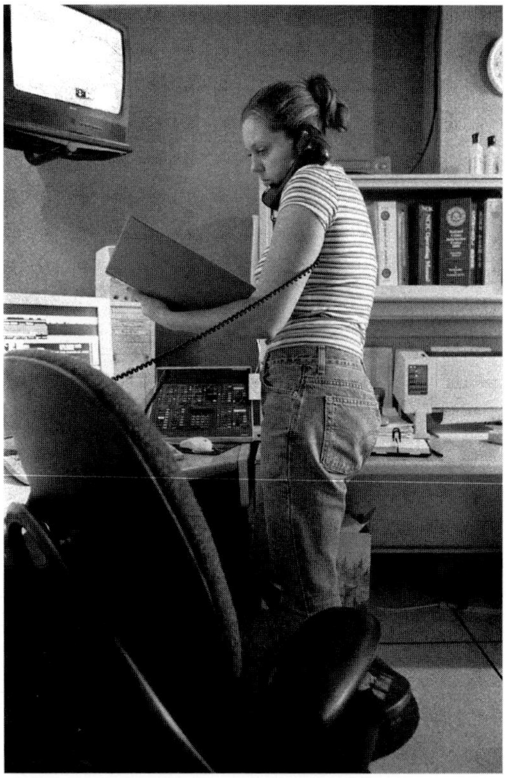

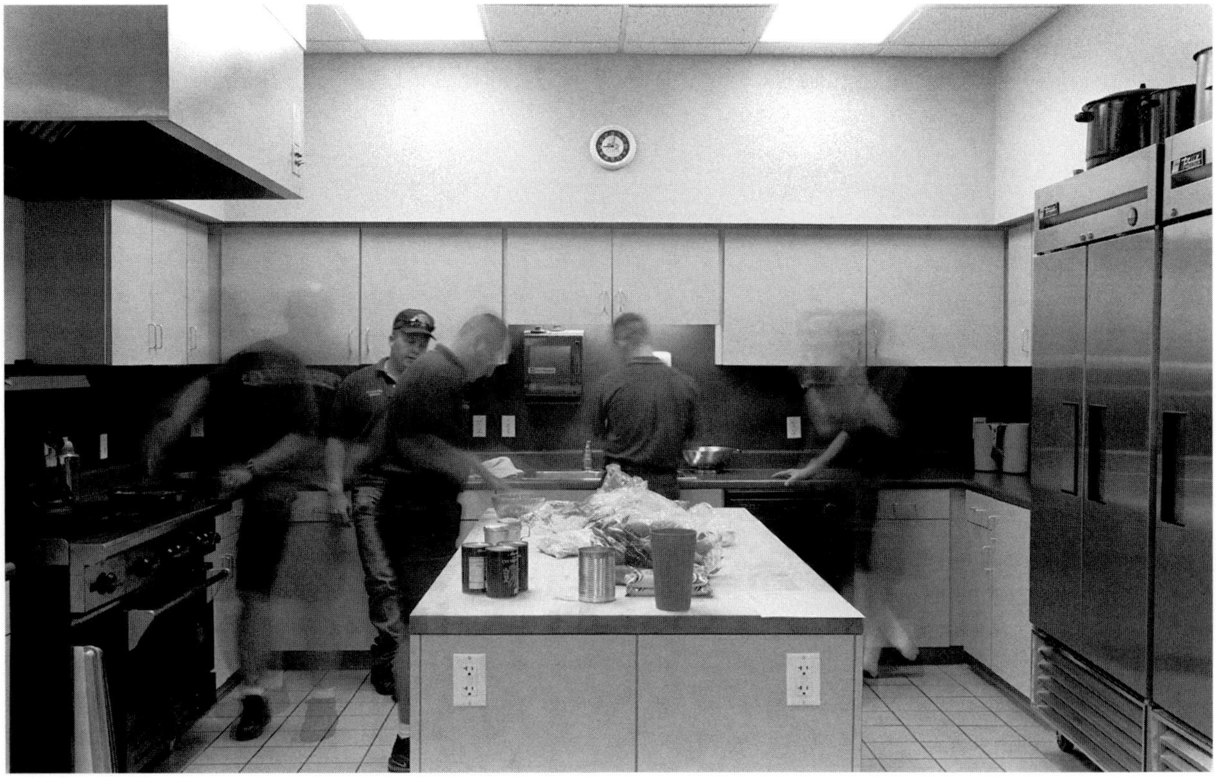

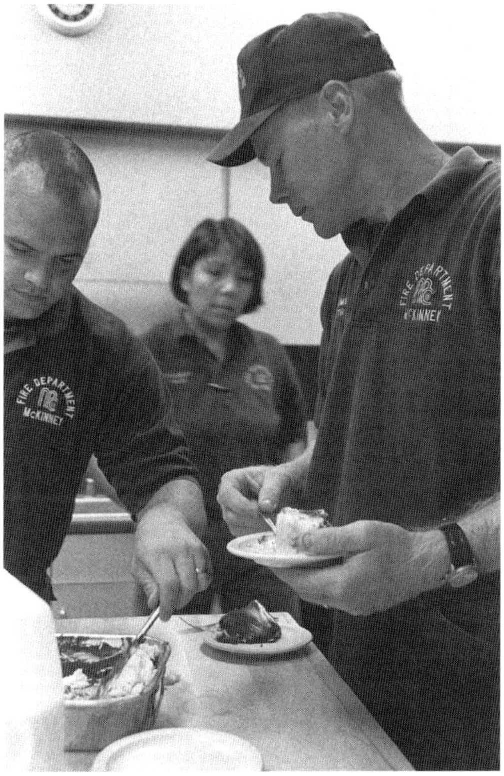
FIRE DEPARTMENT
McKINNEY
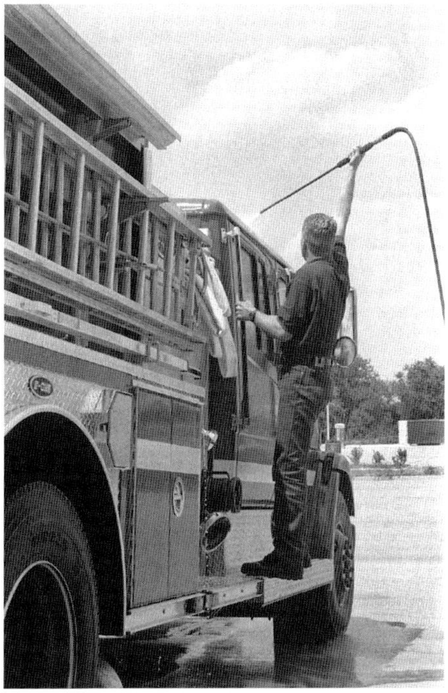
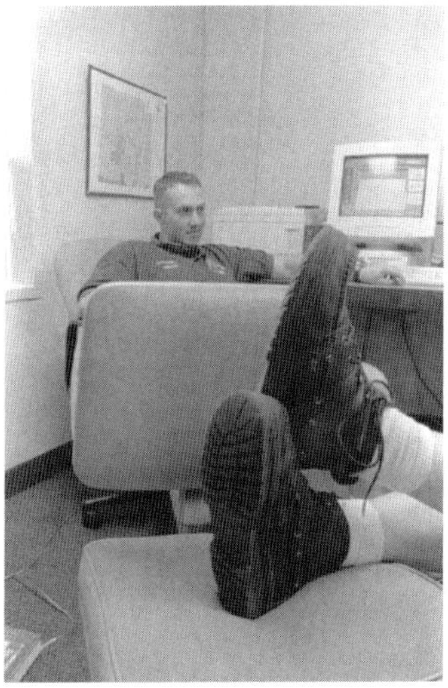
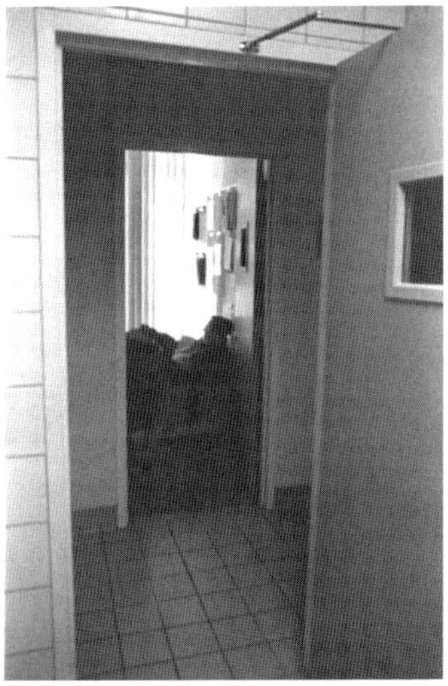
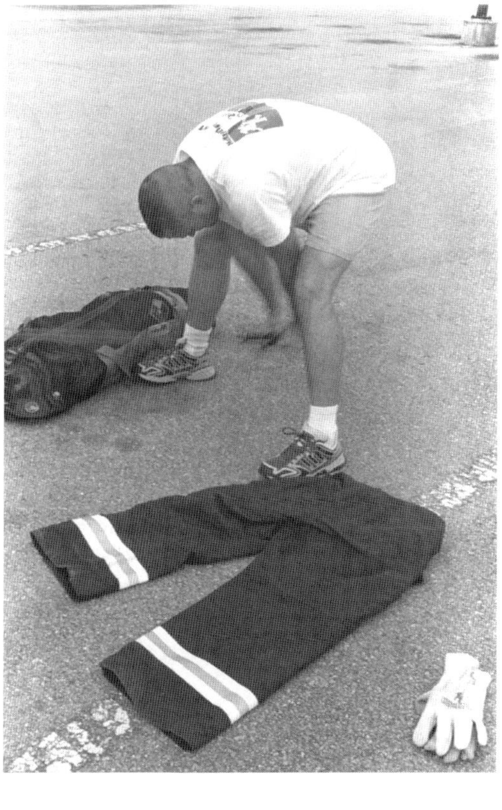

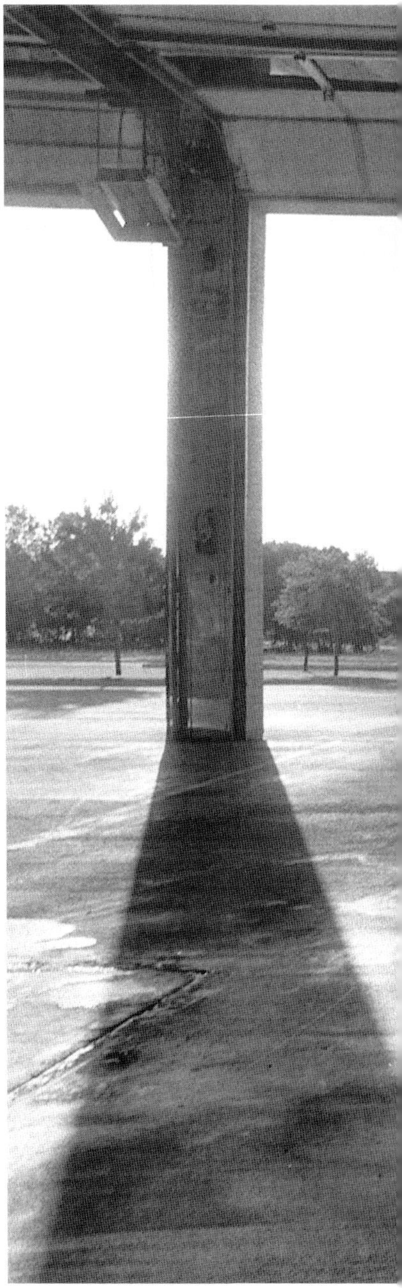

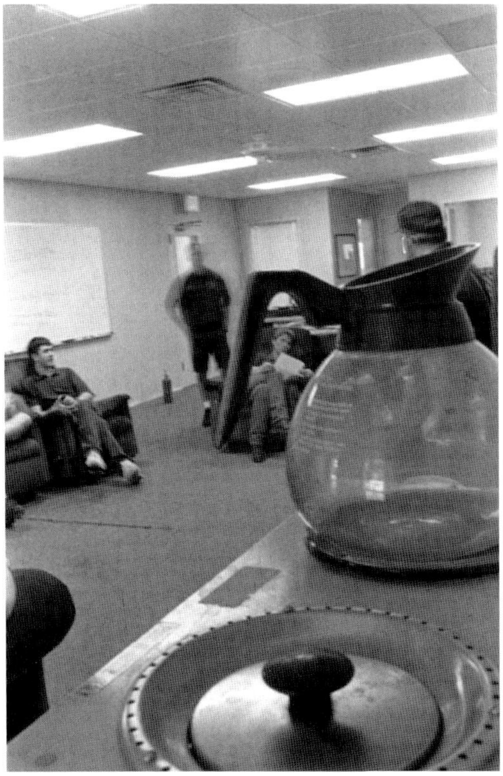

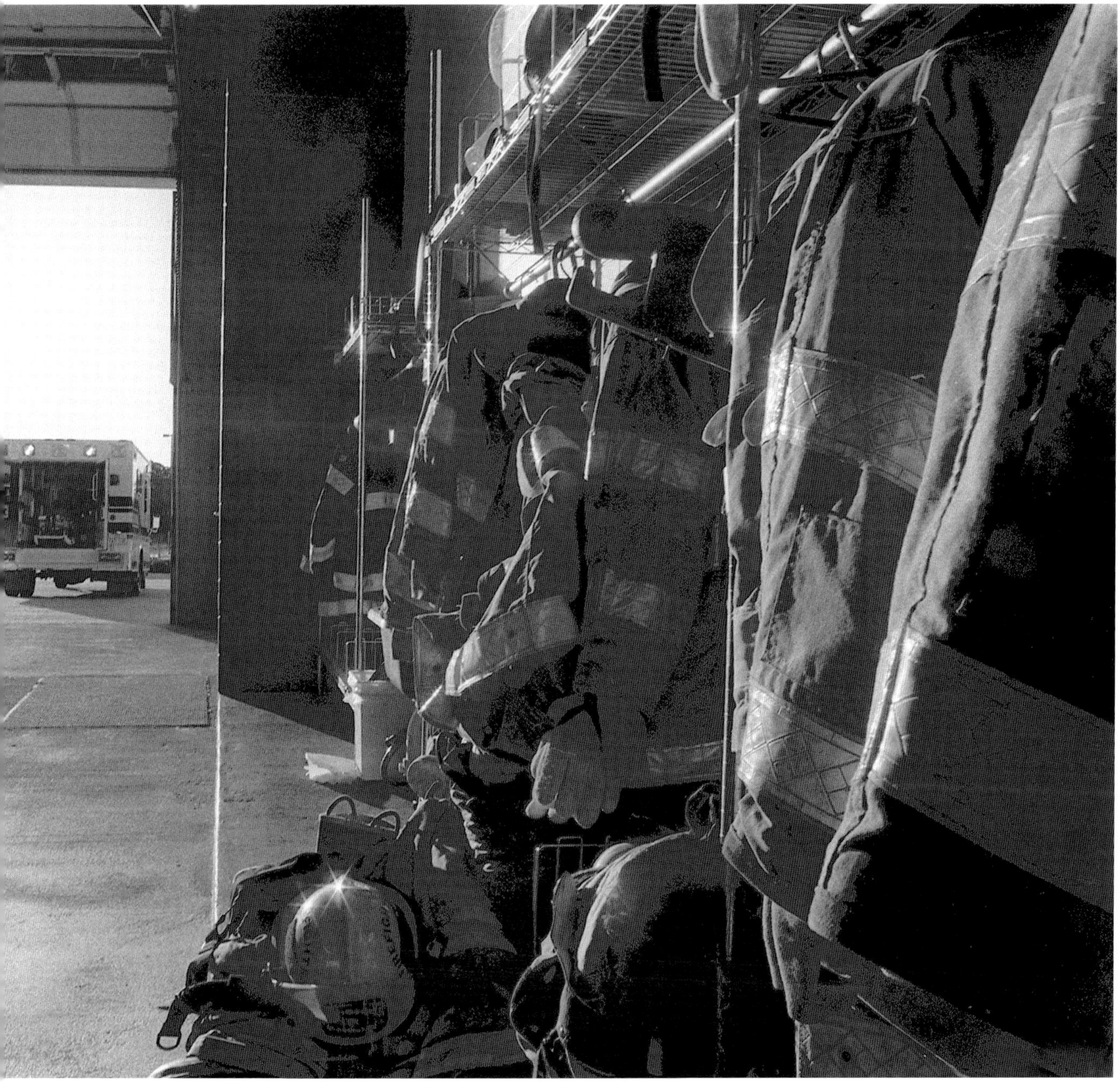

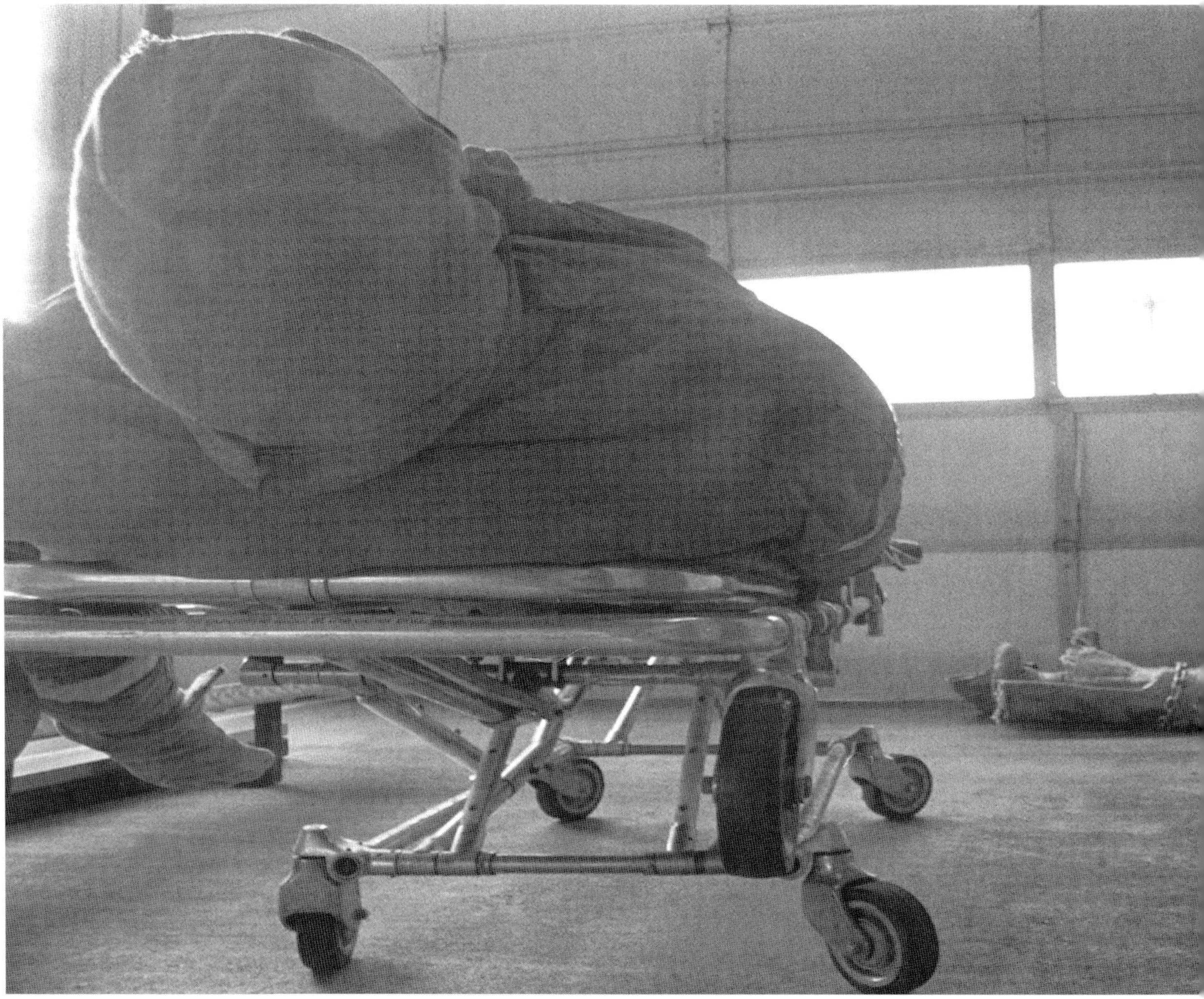

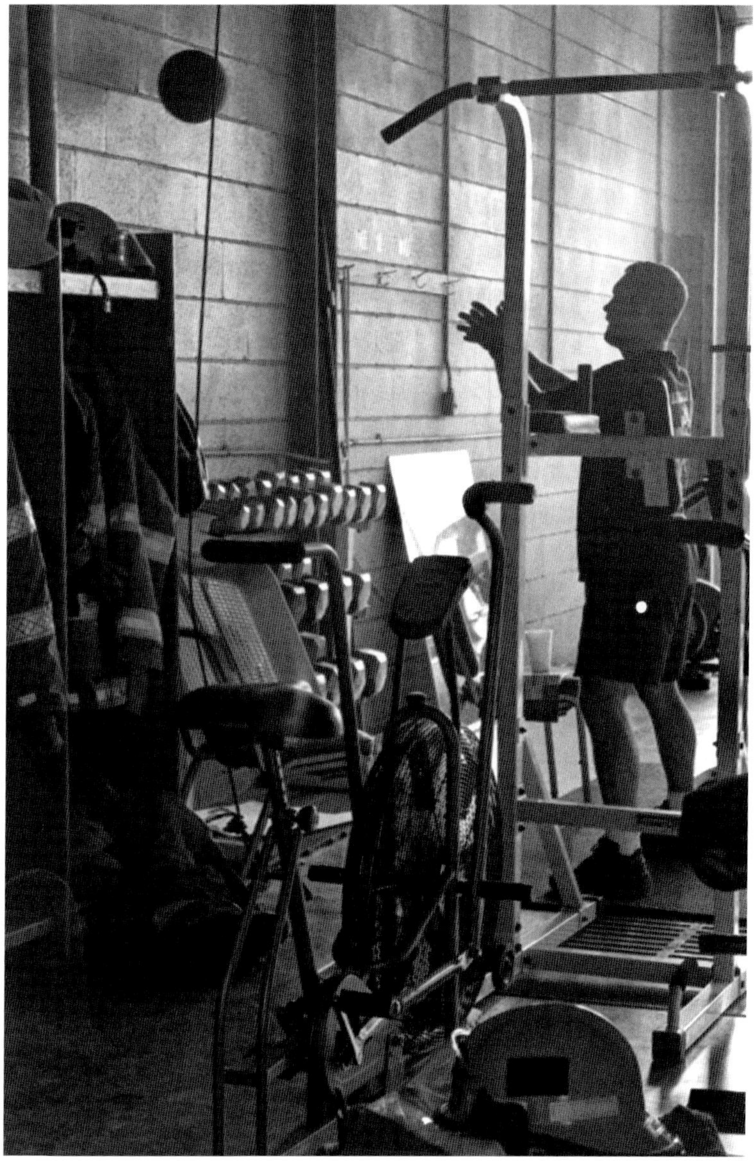

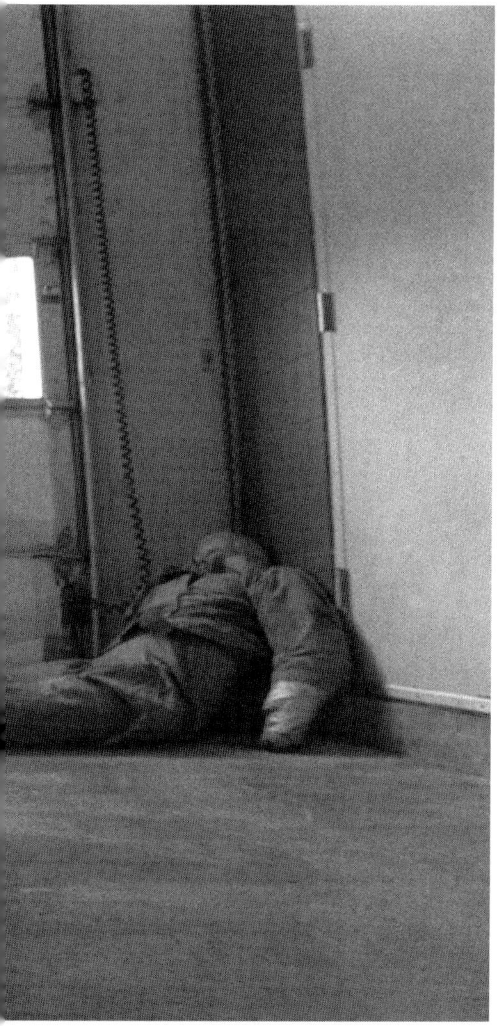

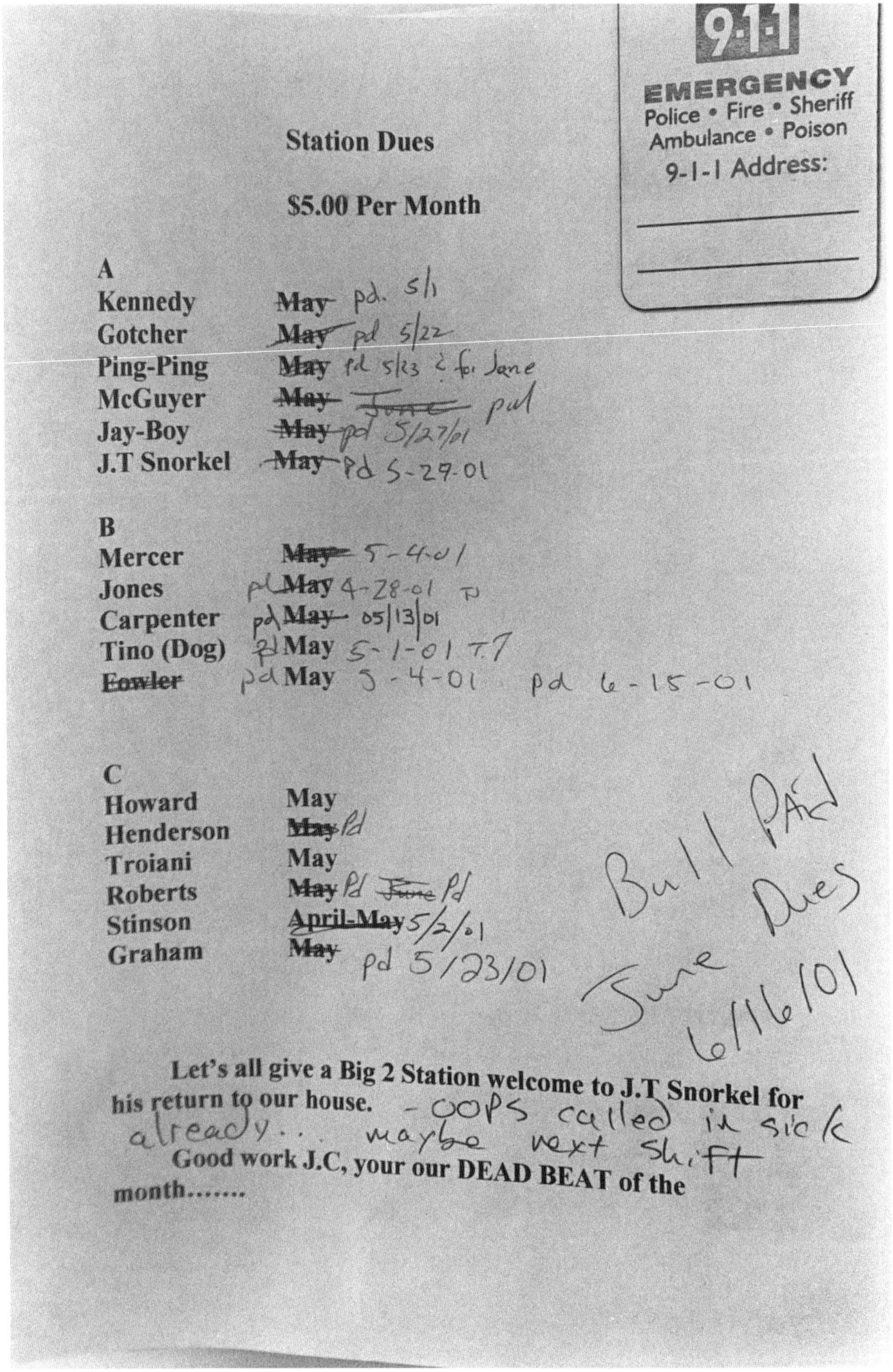



**Station Dues**

**$5.00 Per Month**

**A**
**Kennedy** ~~May~~ pd. 5/1
**Gotcher** ~~May~~ pd 5/22
**Ping-Ping** ~~May~~ pd 5/23 & for June
**McGuyer** ~~May~~ ~~June~~ pd
**Jay-Boy** ~~May~~ pd 5/27/01
**J.T Snorkel** ~~May~~ Pd 5-27-01

**B**
**Mercer** ~~May~~ 5-4-01
**Jones** pd ~~May~~ 4-28-01 TJ
**Carpenter** pd ~~May~~ 05/13/01
**Tino (Dog)** pd May 5-1-01 TJ
~~**Fowler**~~ pd May 5-4-01 pd 6-15-01

**C**
**Howard** May
**Henderson** ~~May~~ Pd
**Troiani** May
**Roberts** ~~May~~ Pd ~~June~~ Pd
**Stinson** ~~April-May~~ 5/2/01
**Graham** ~~May~~ pd 5/23/01

Bull PAid June Dues 6/16/01

**Let's all give a Big 2 Station welcome to J.T Snorkel for his return to our house.** - OOPS called in sick already.. maybe next shift

**Good work J.C, your our DEAD BEAT of the month.......**

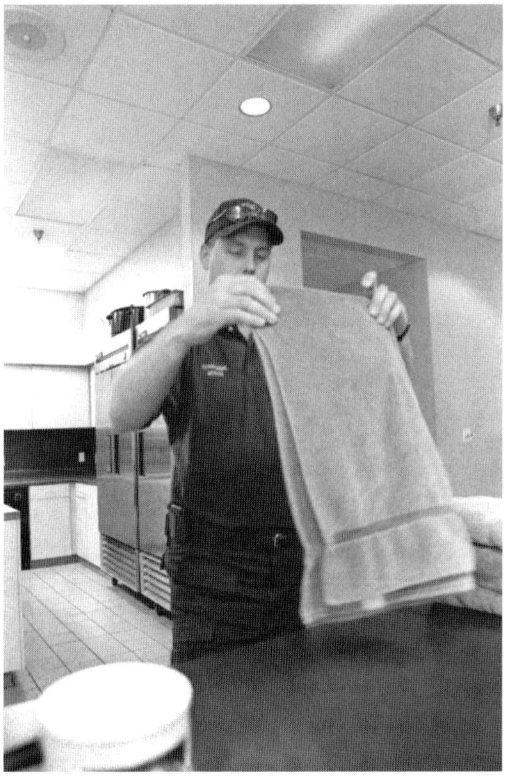

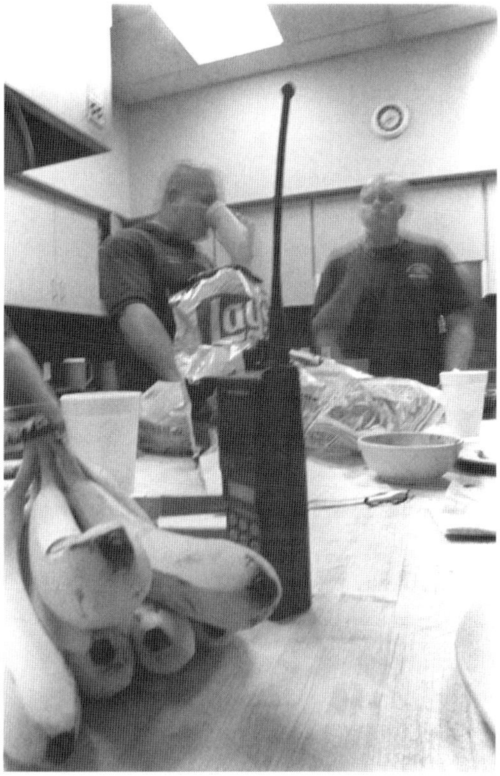

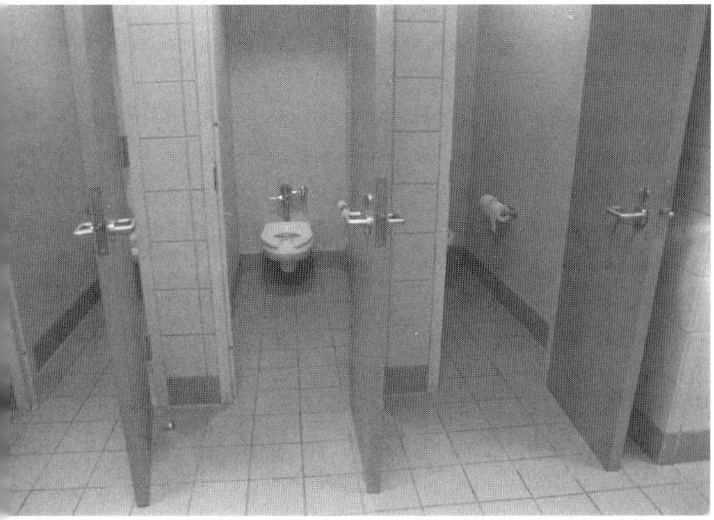

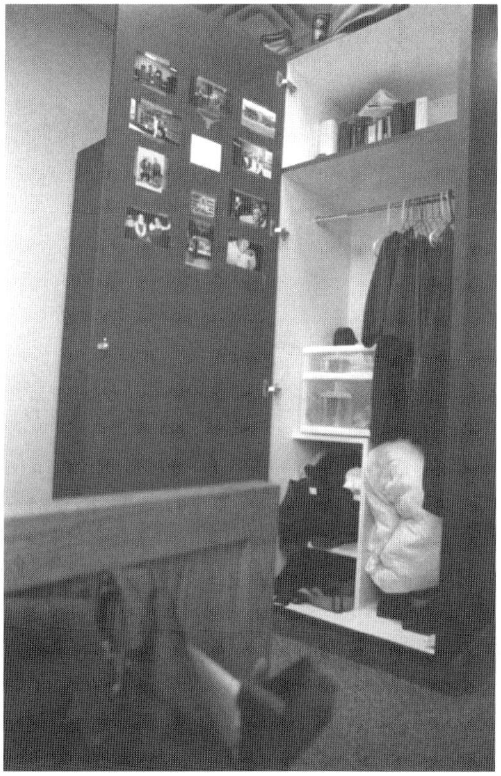

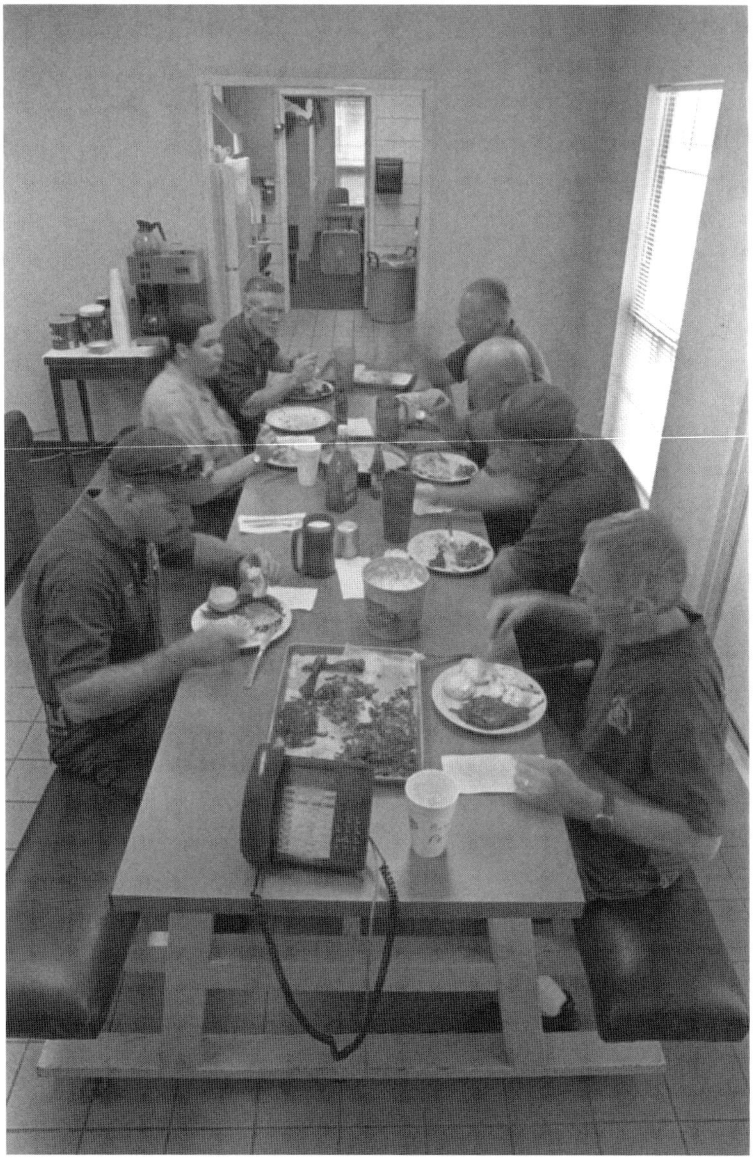

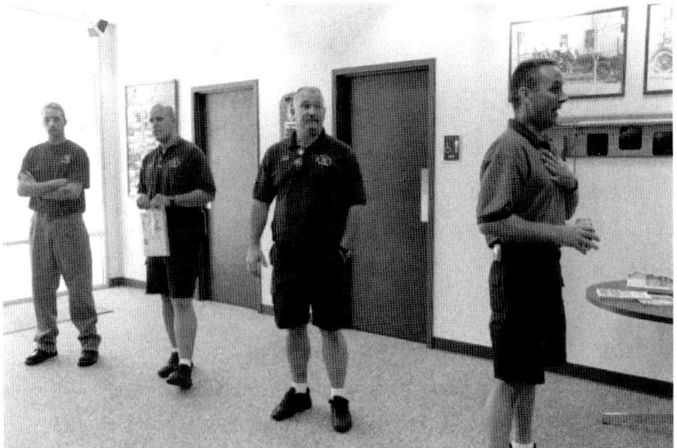

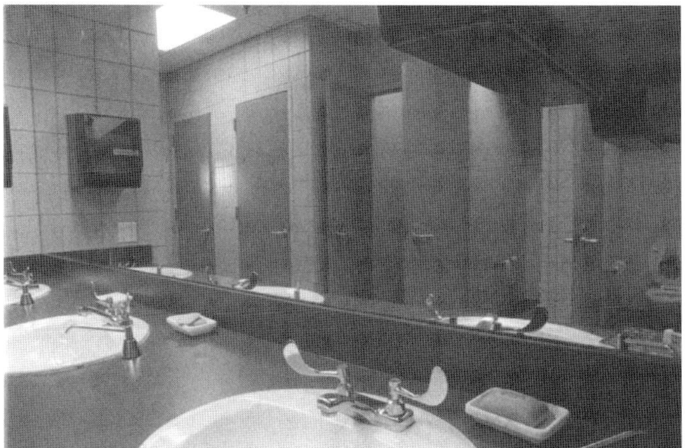

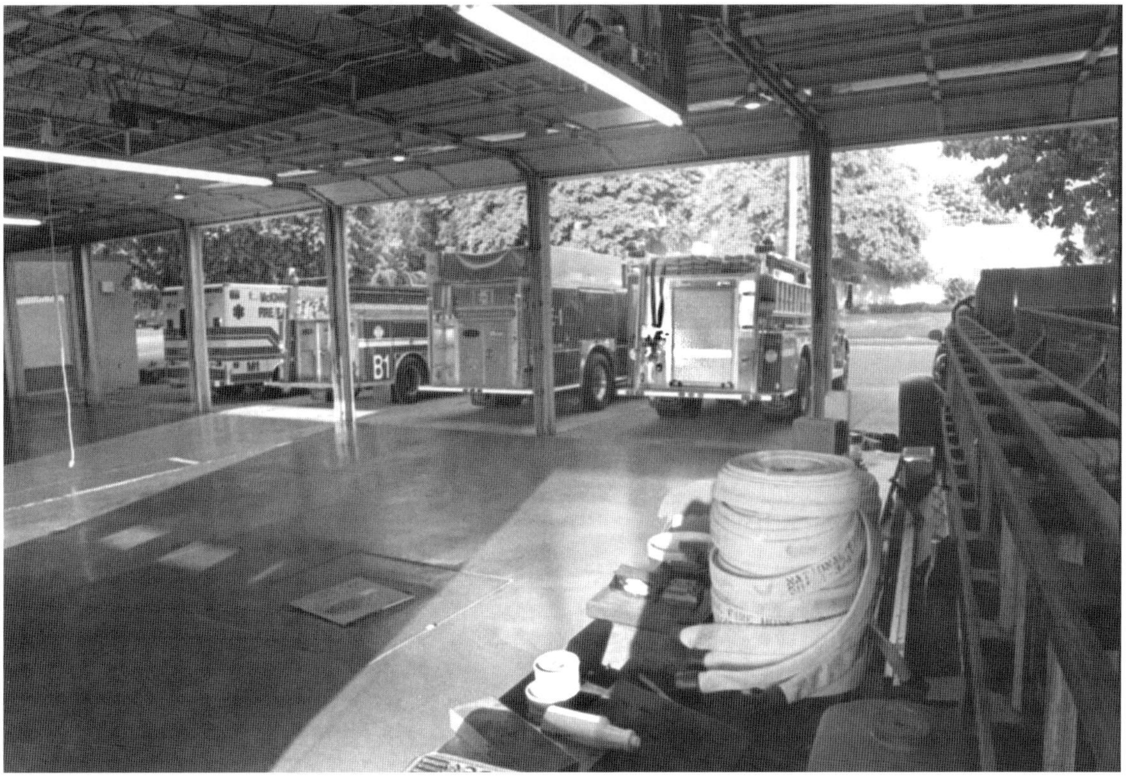
B1

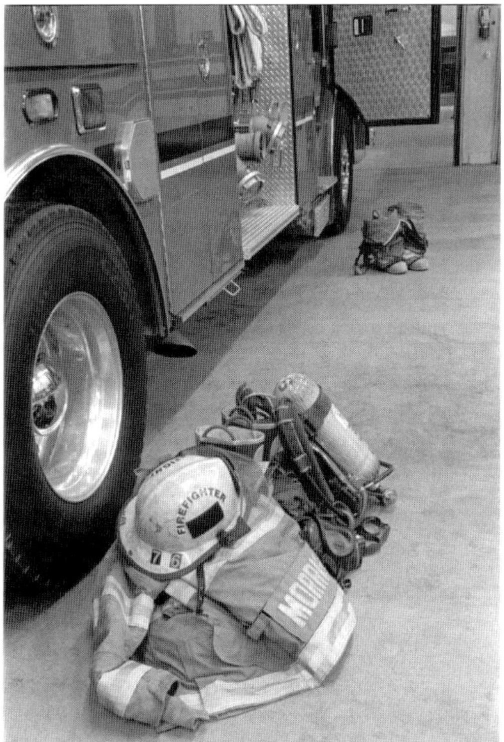
FIREFIGHTER
76

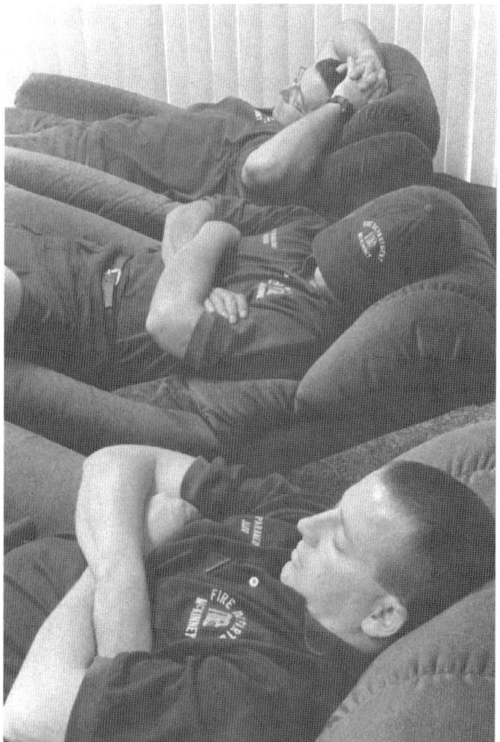

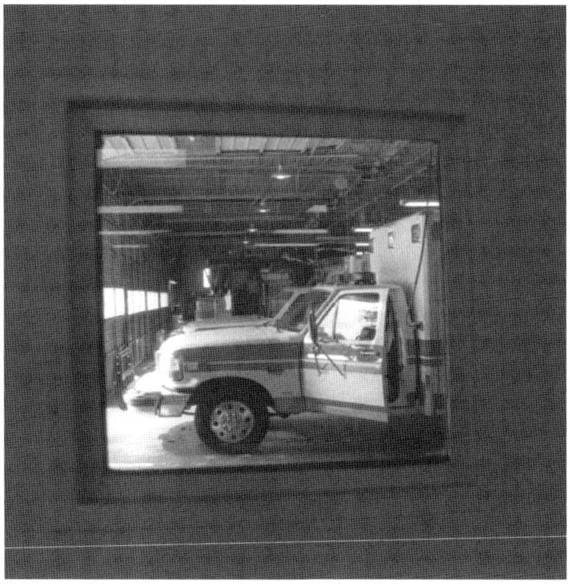

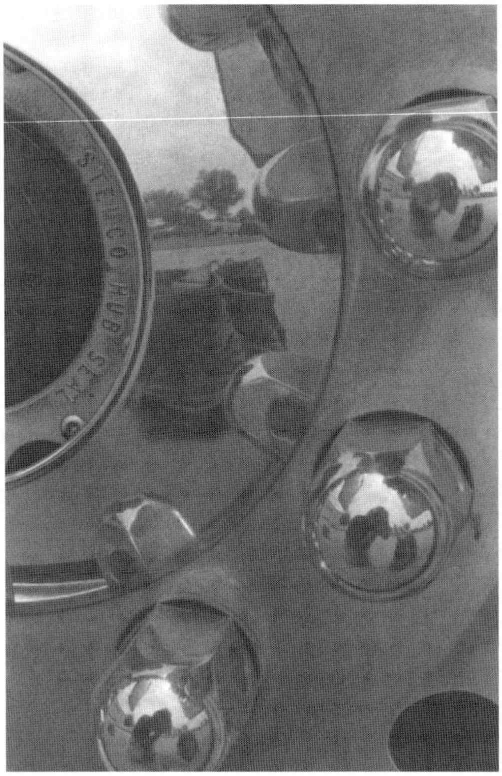

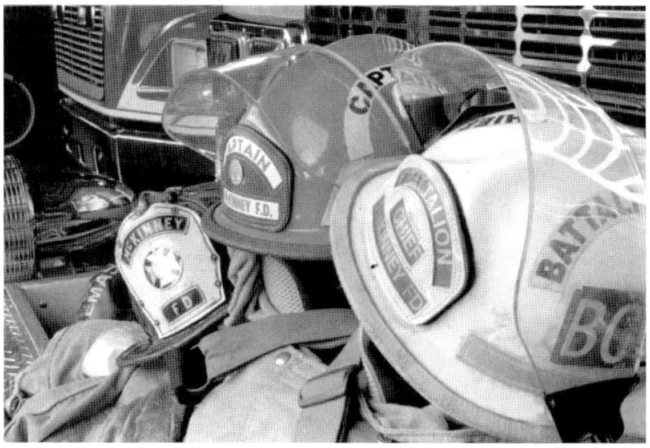
McKINNEY
FD

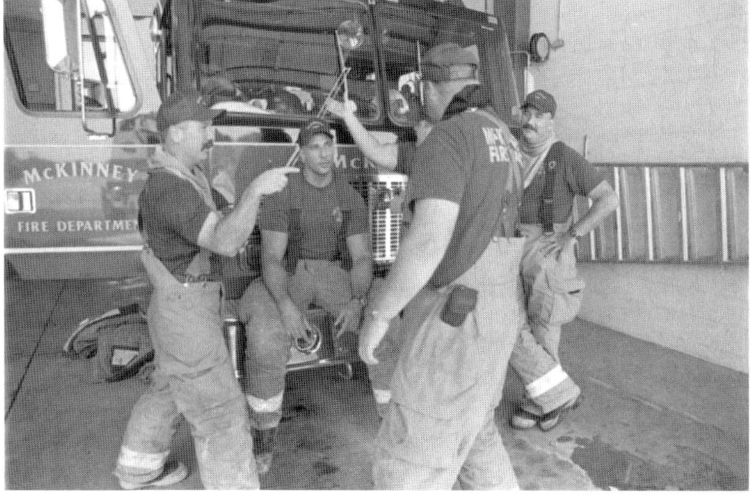
McKINNEY

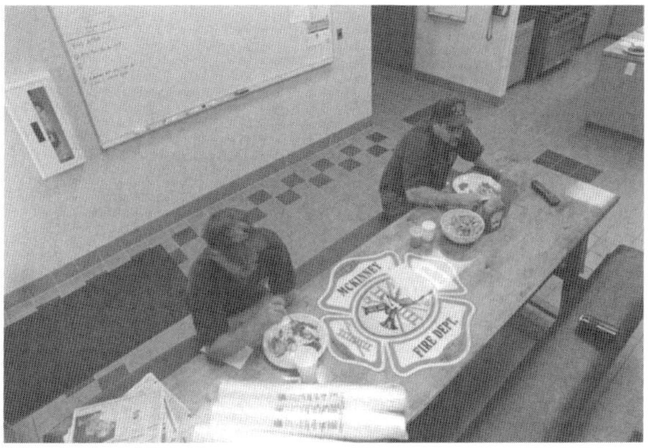
McKINNEY
FIRE DEPT.

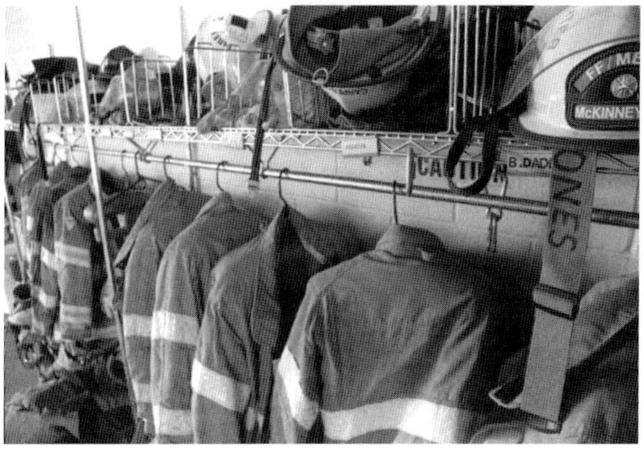
McKINNEY
CAUTION

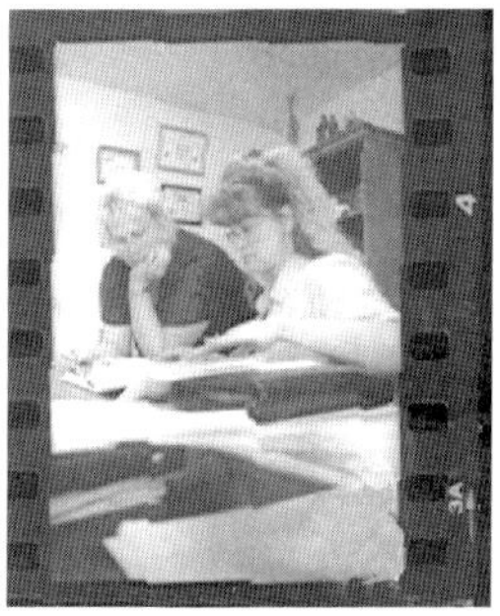

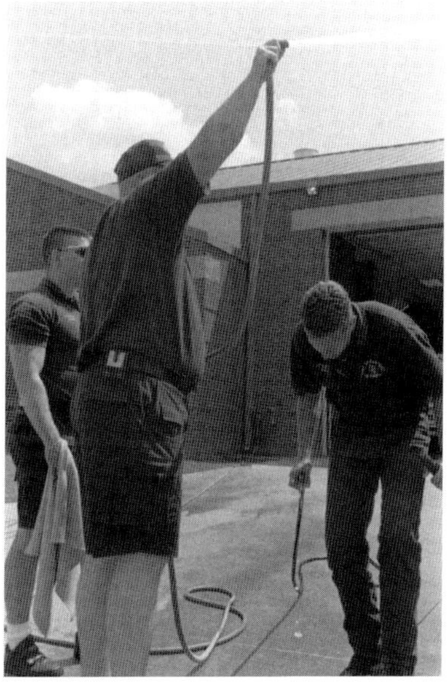

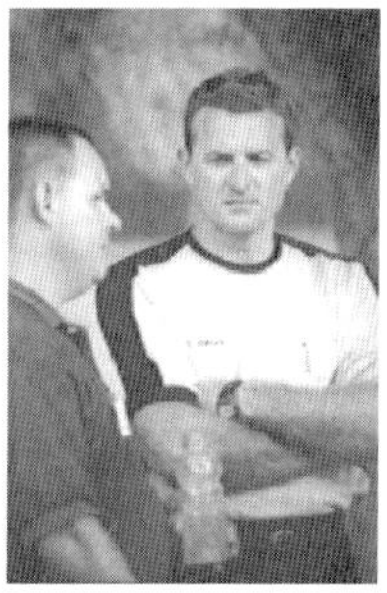

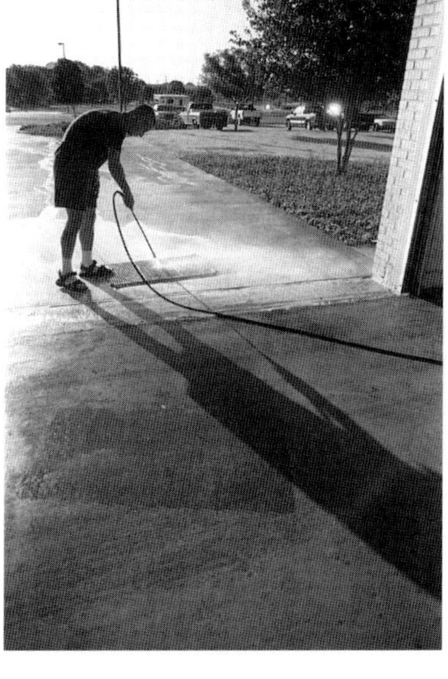

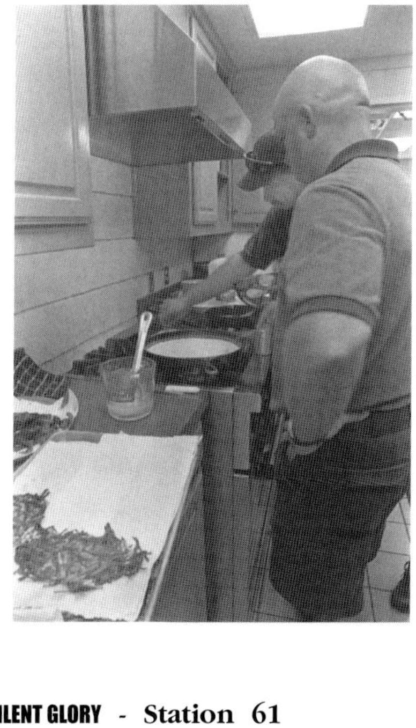

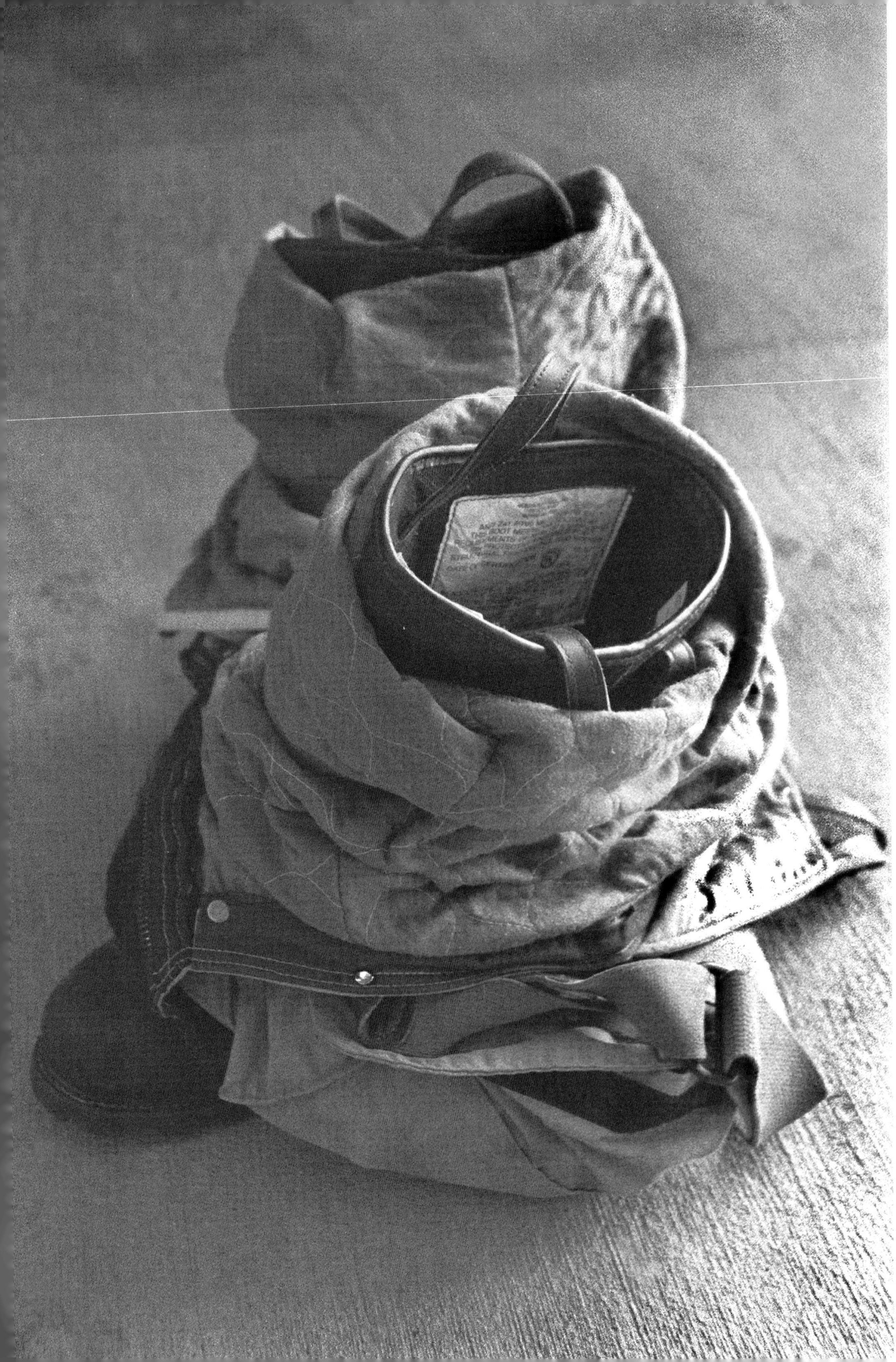

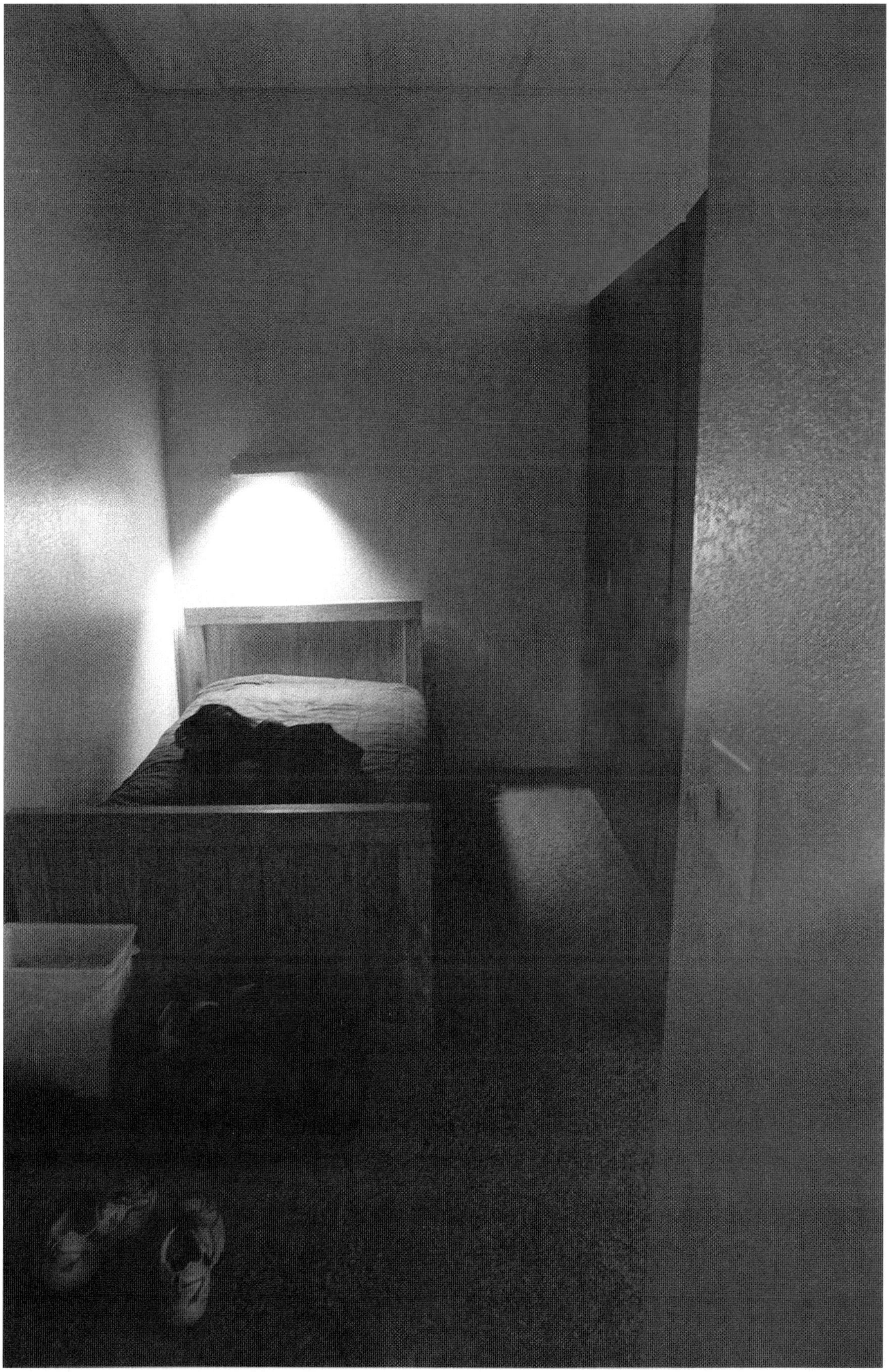

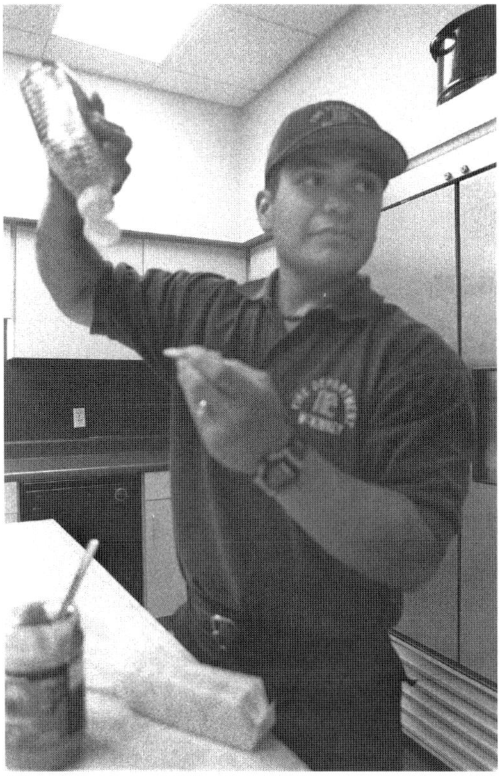

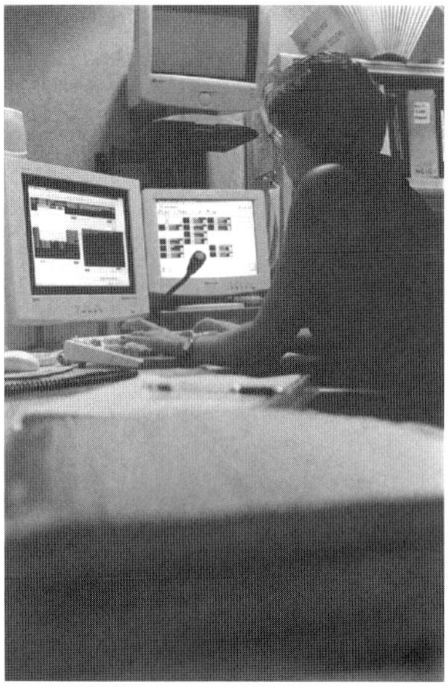

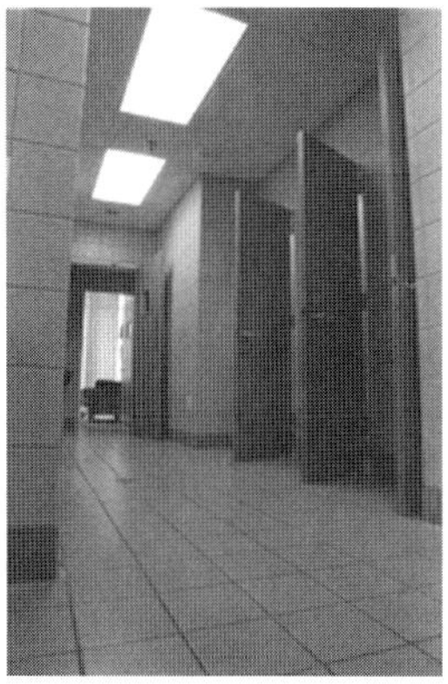

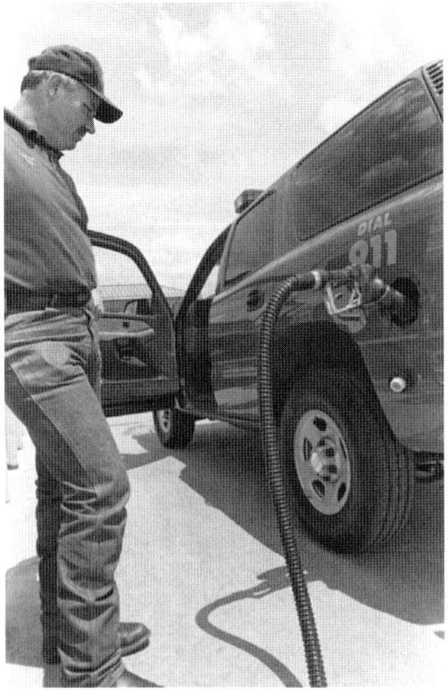
DIAL
911

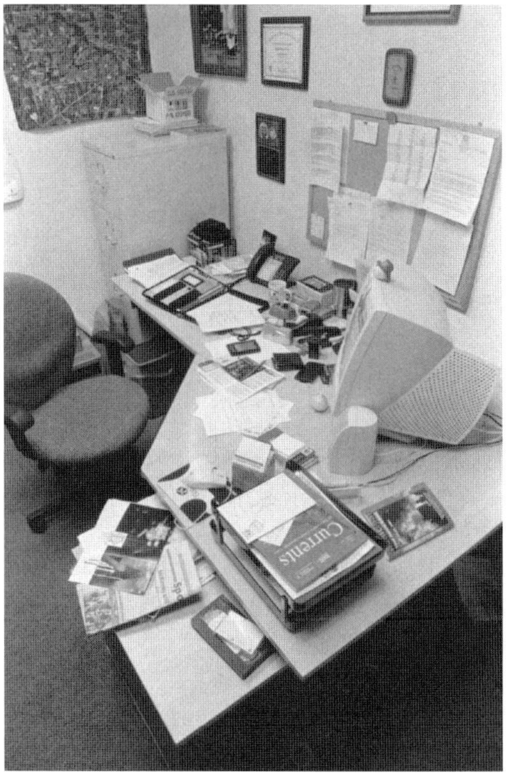

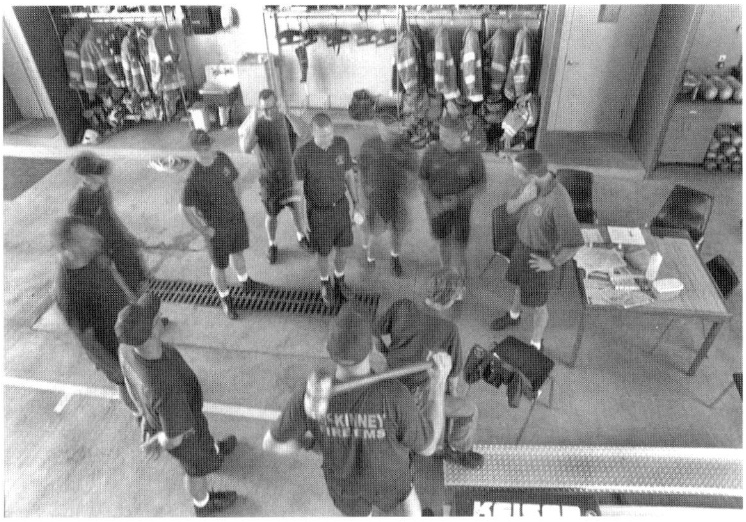

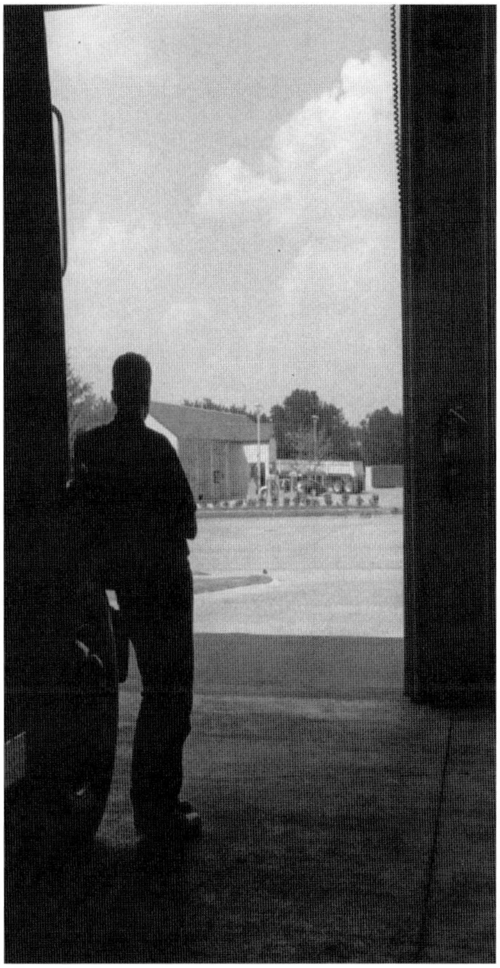

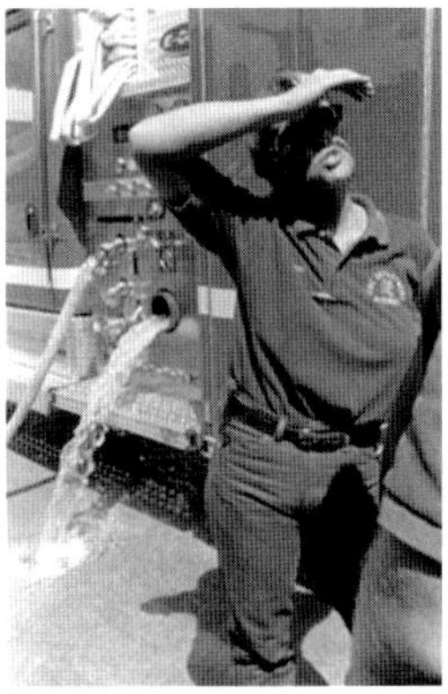

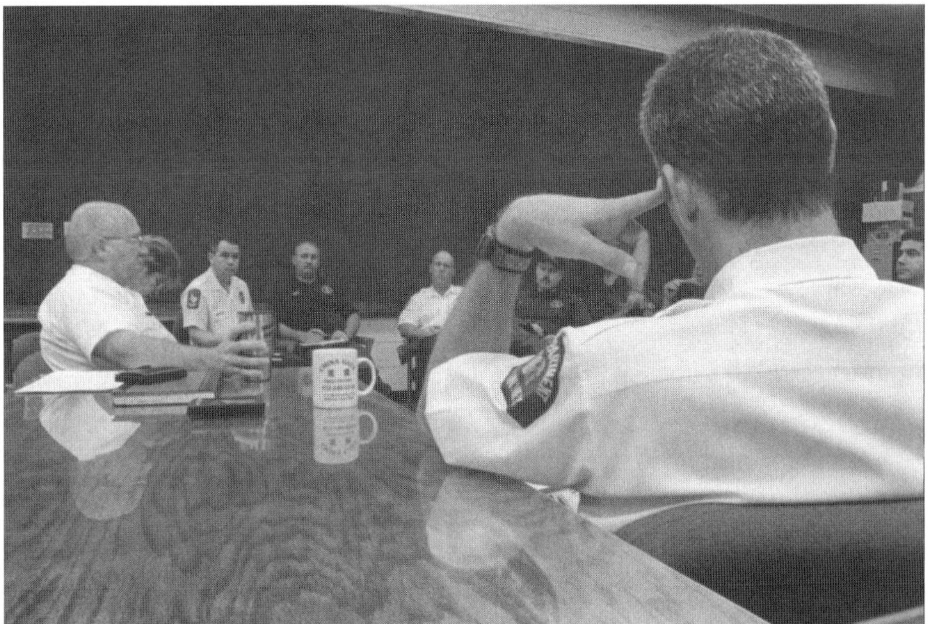

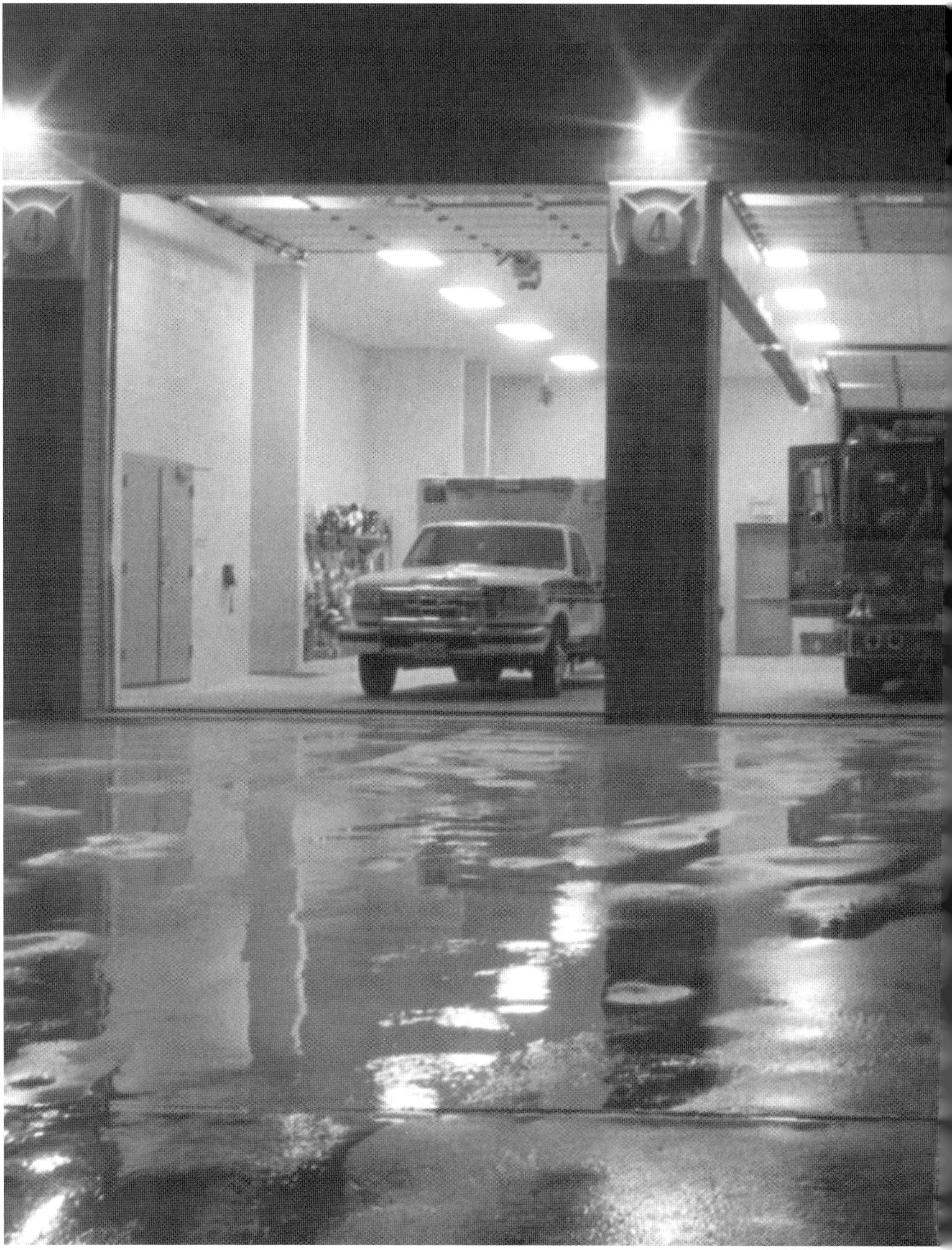

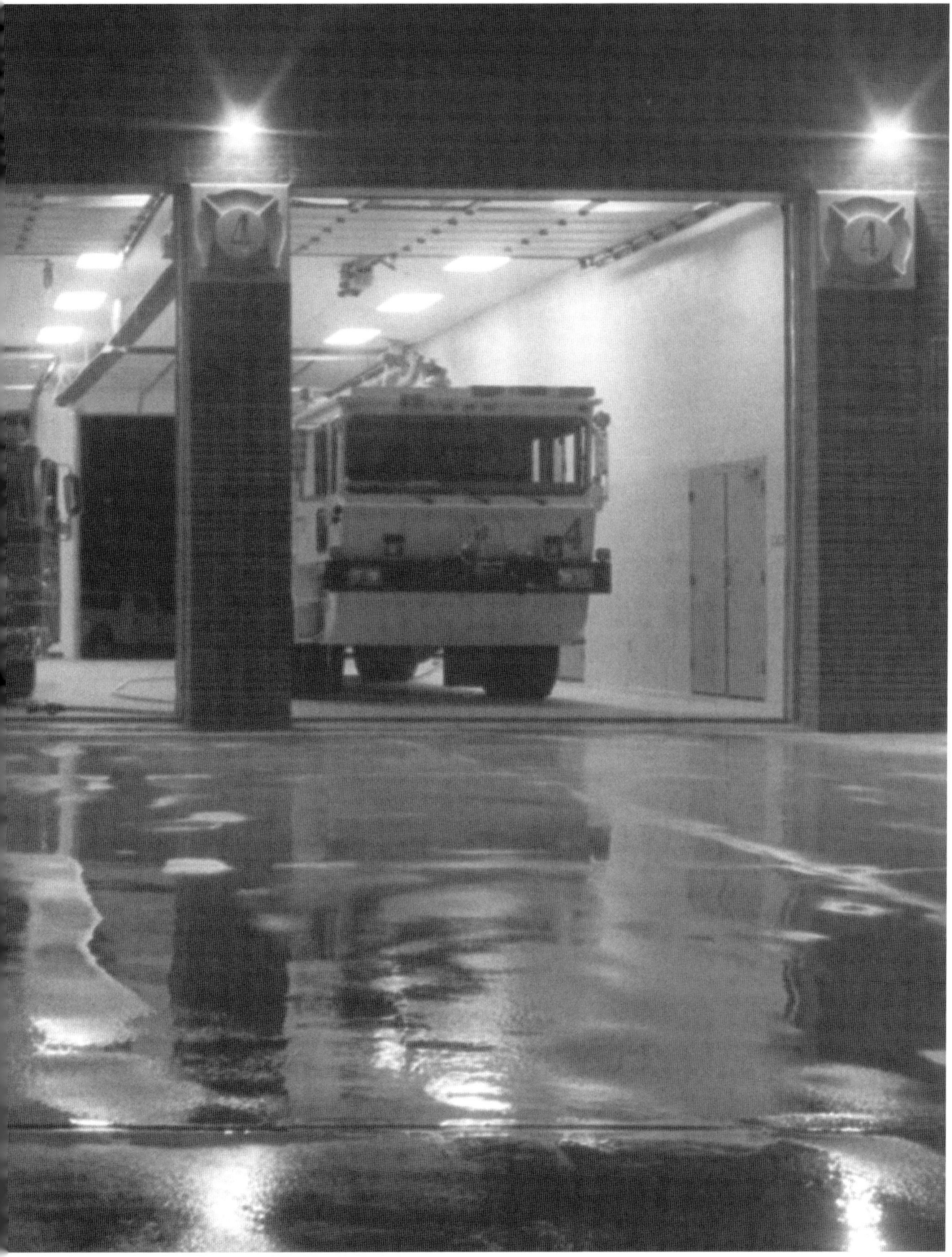

# medical

Times change, things change. Because of mobile medical technology advances, most fire departments acquired emergency or paramedic care responsibilities in addition to fire fighting. It was a natural. So much so that medical calls now typically represent 75% of all calls in a combined Fire/EMS Department.

Most times when a call comes in for emergency medical service, a fire engine goes along with the ambulance, just in case... Ever carry a 350 lb. bedridden down several flights of stairs? No? Well, you can use every available hand to do so. Or, when it is an unexpected early delivery, it's always nice to have a cheering section nearby for the mom and the EMS/paramedic folks who are assisting her.

Today's Firefighters are typically certificated not only in fire fighting but also emergency medical technology and/or paramedicine. When time counts, they do it, and don't have to wait around for someone else to show up. Makes sense. Ask all those snatched from the very brink who needed immediate help and action. I know, I am one of them, several times over.

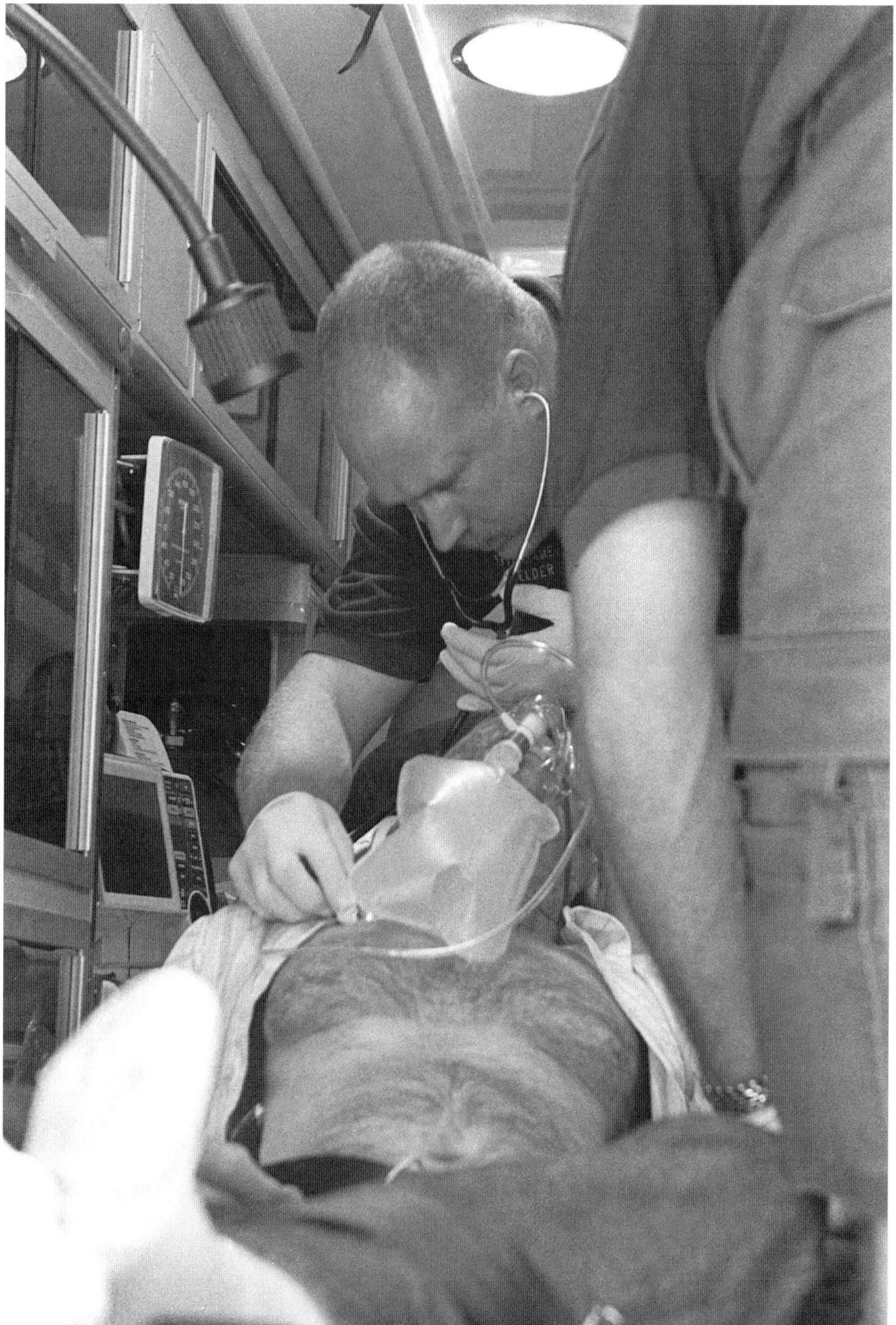

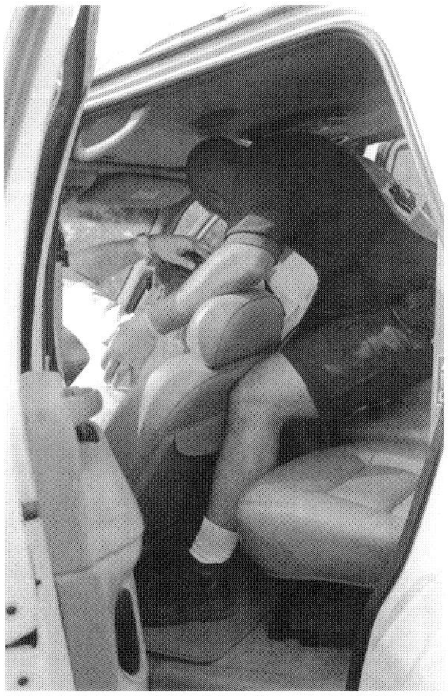

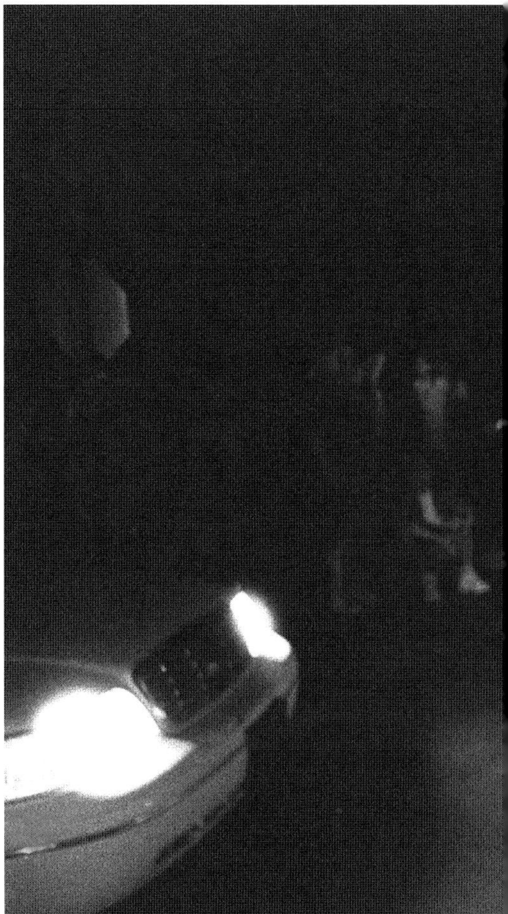

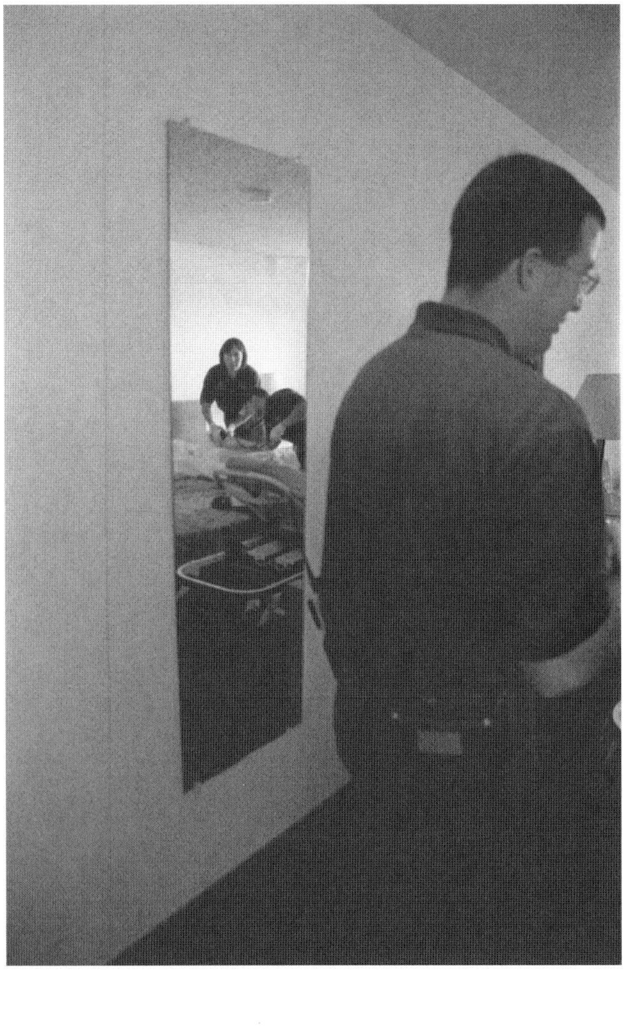

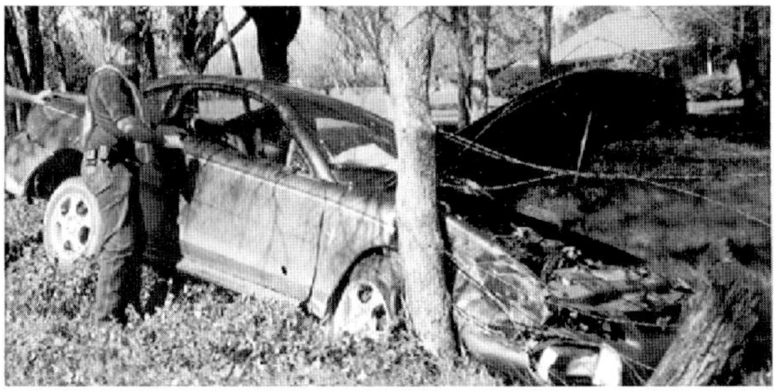

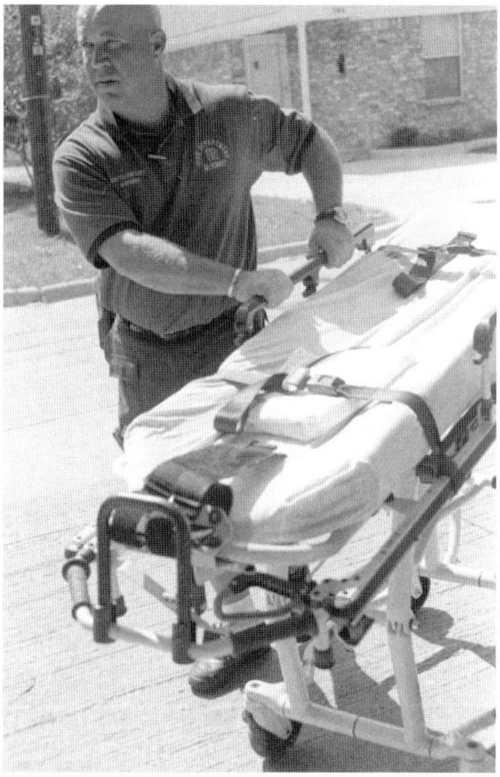

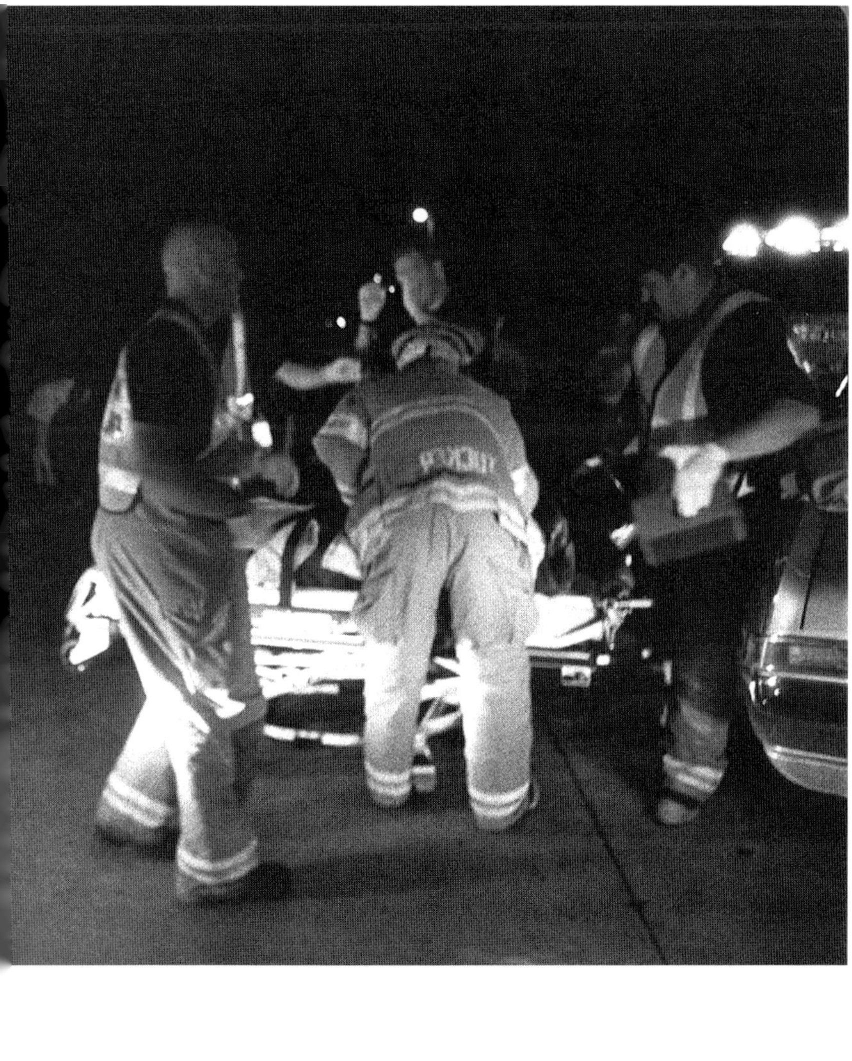

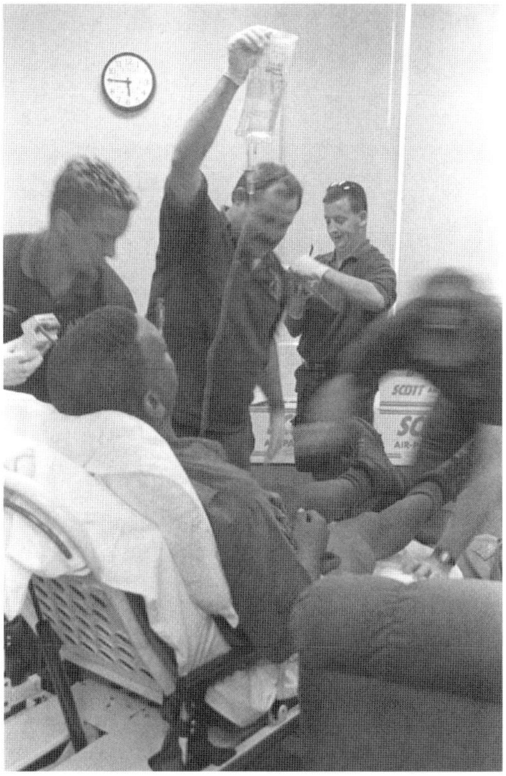

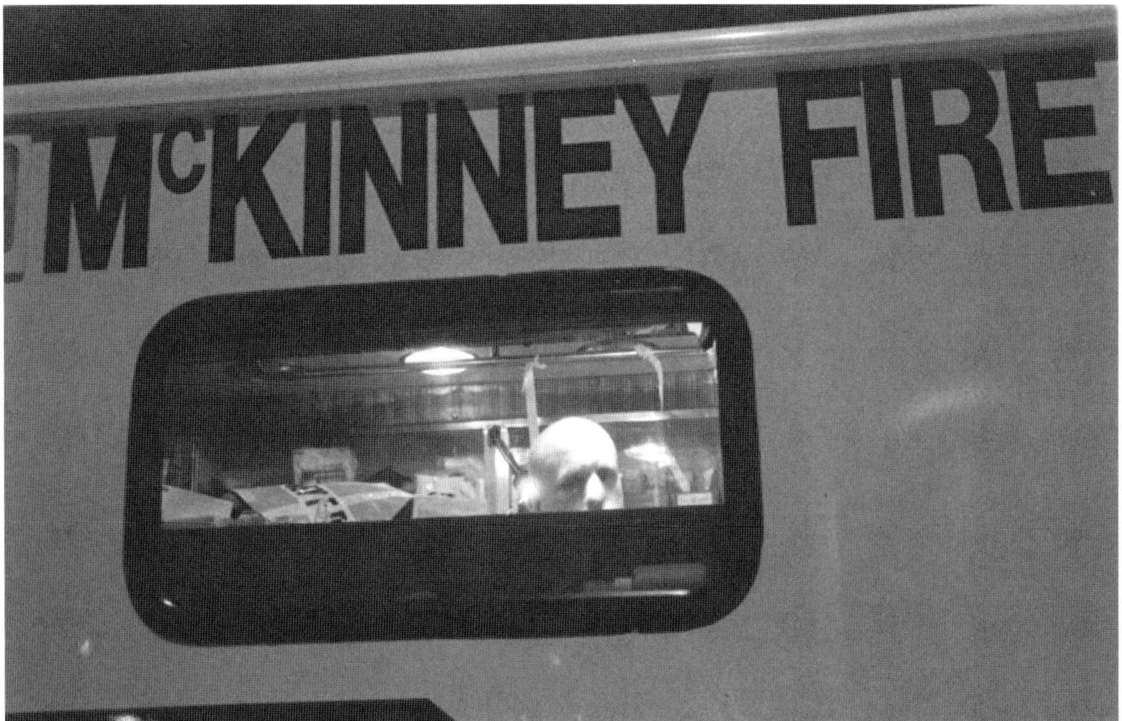
McKINNEY FIRE

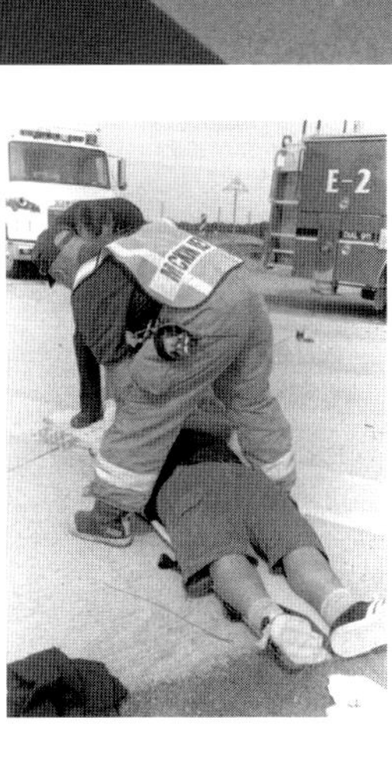
E-2

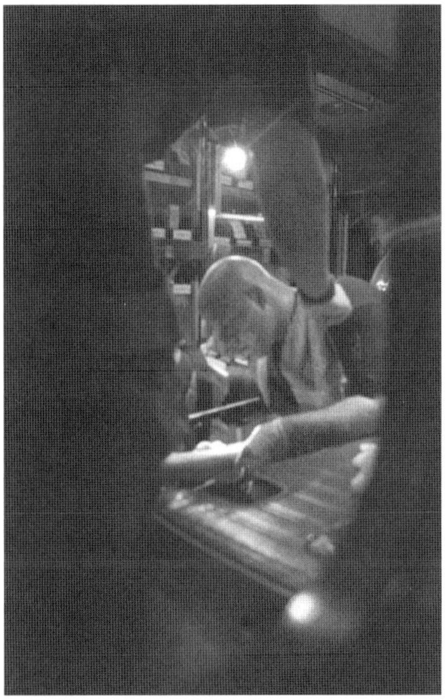

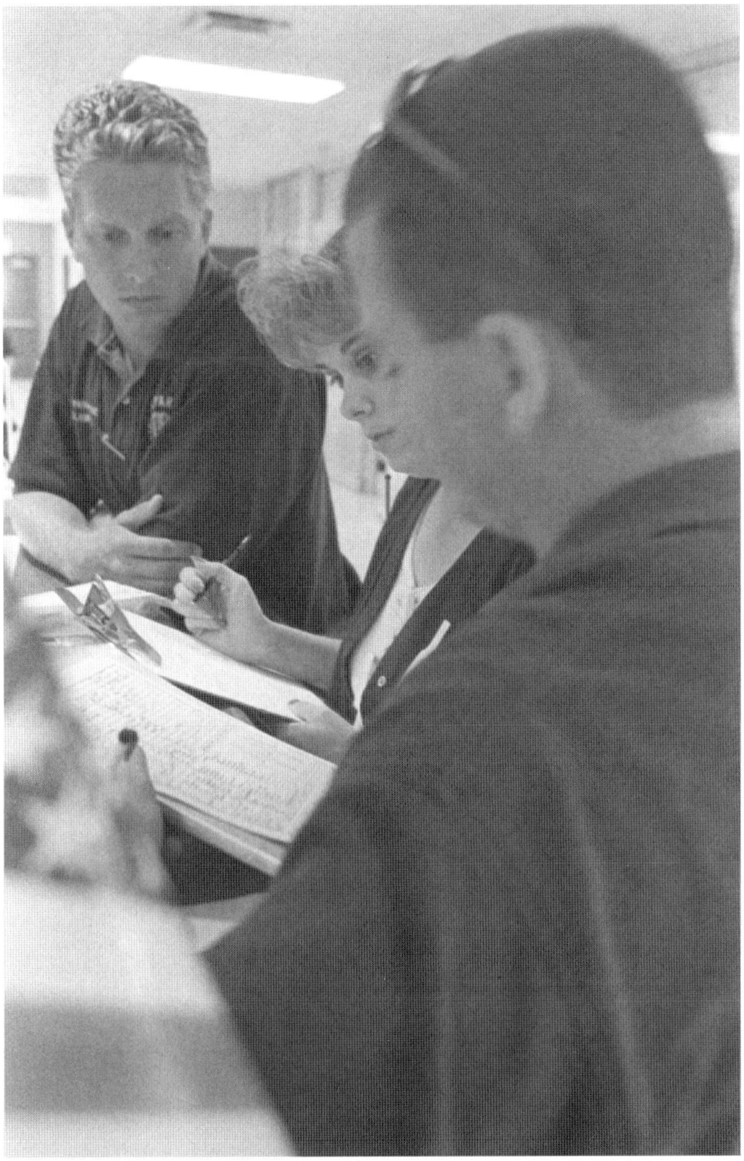

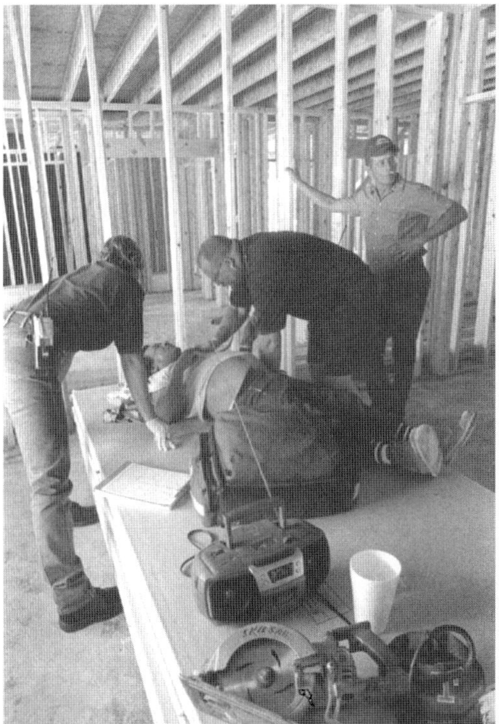

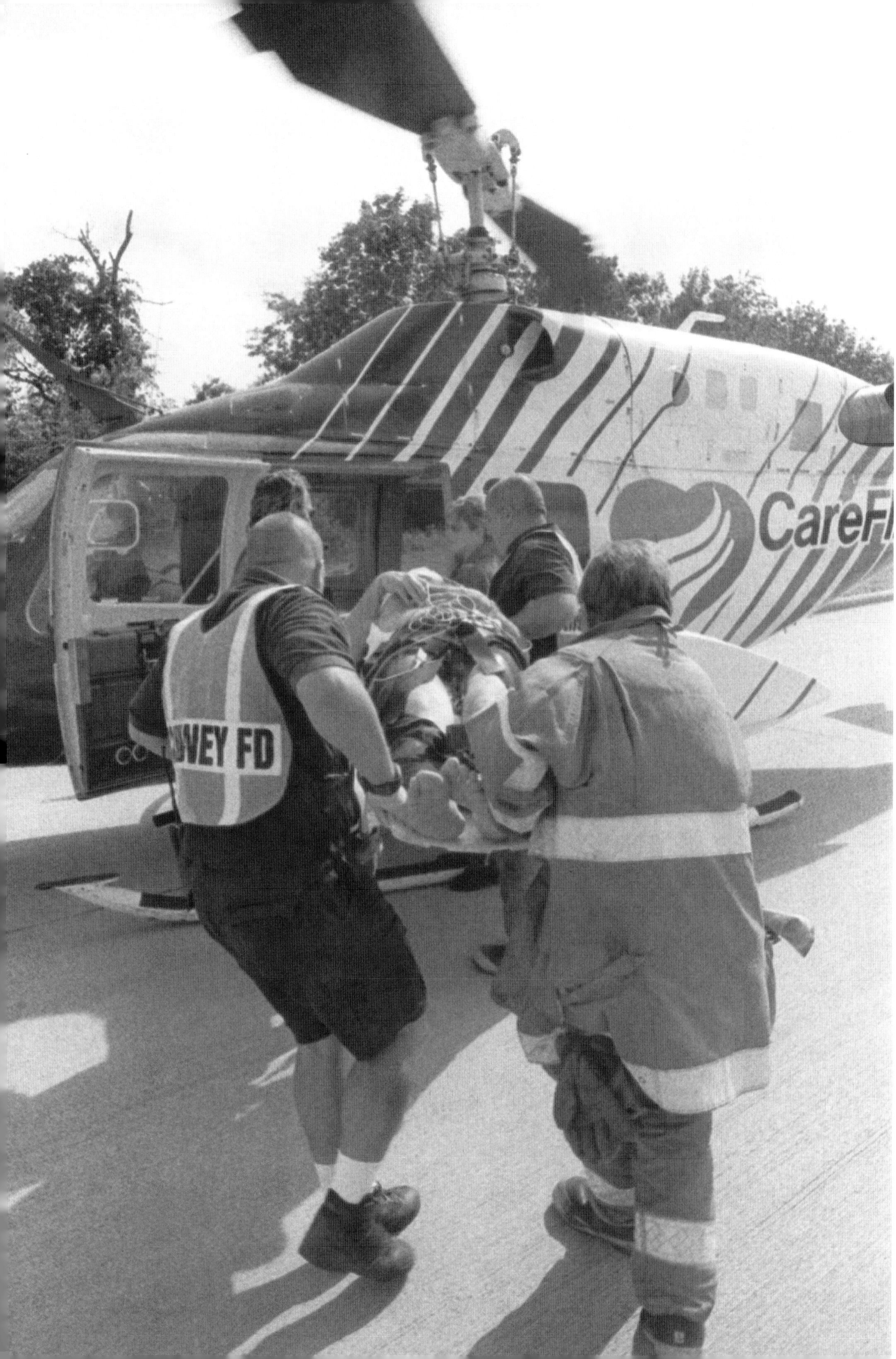

CareFl
VEY FD

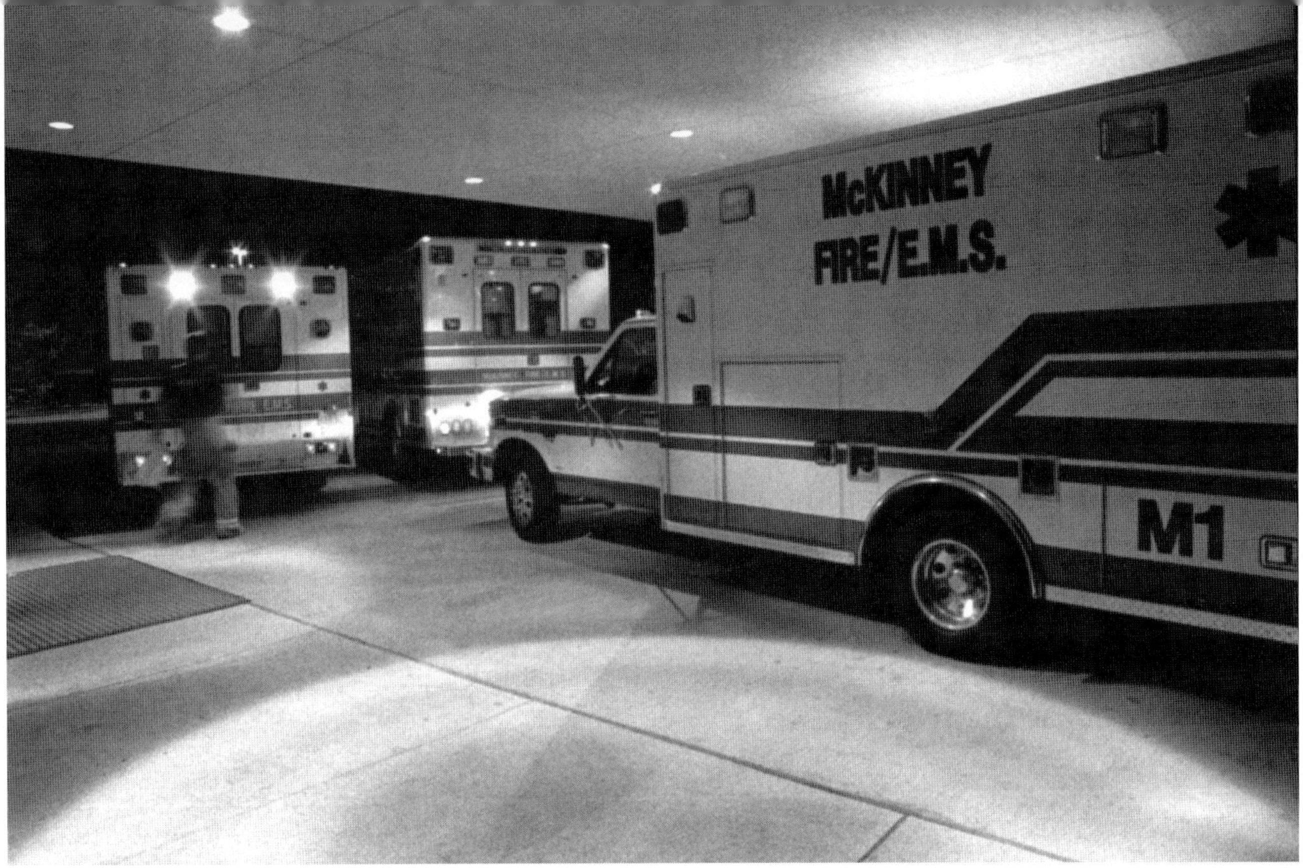
McKINNEY
FIRE/E.M.S.
M1

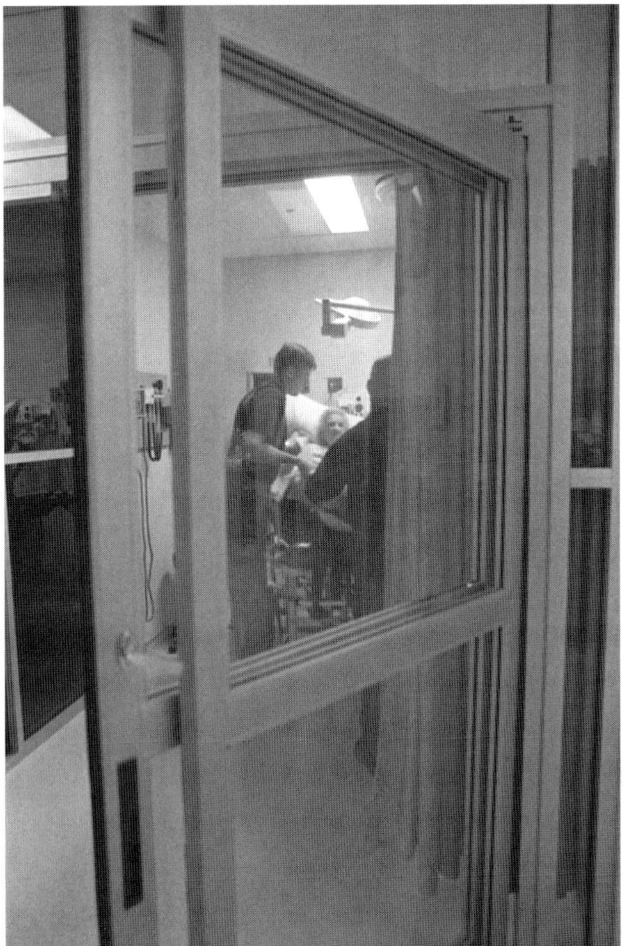

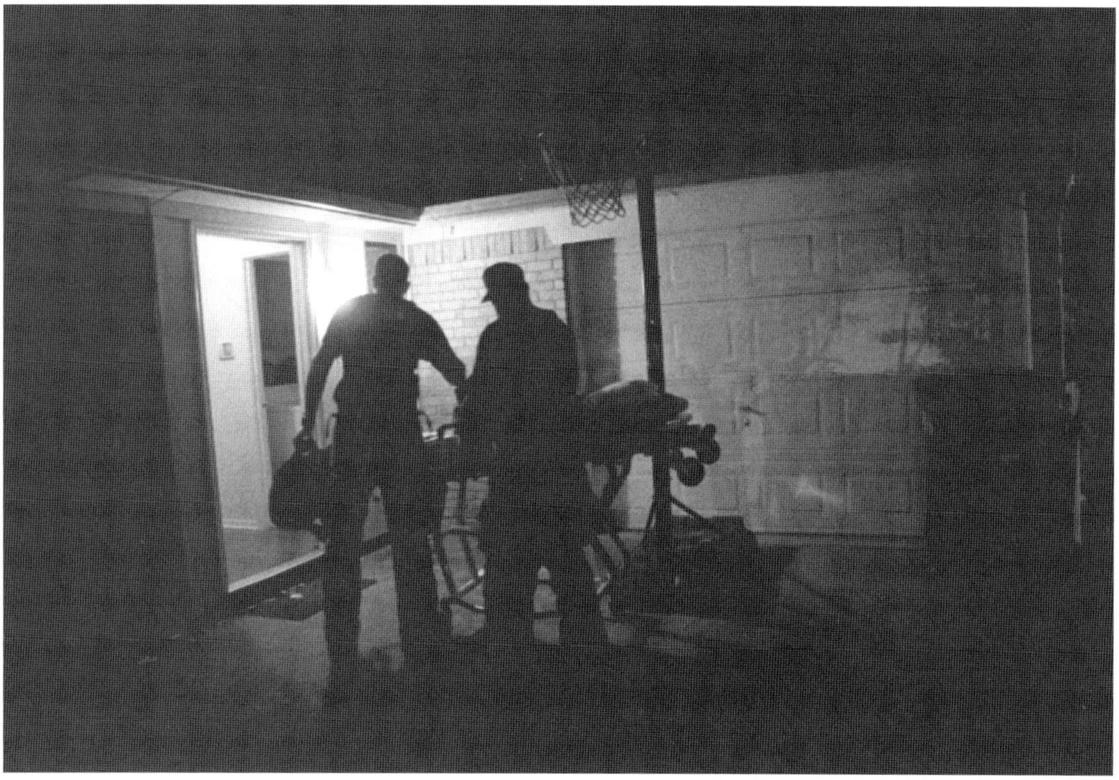

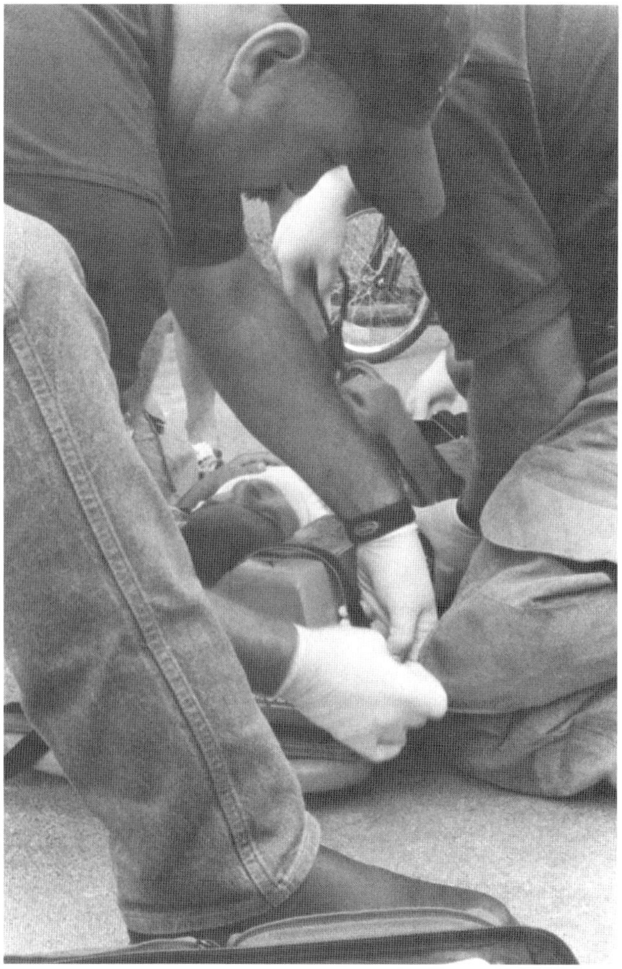

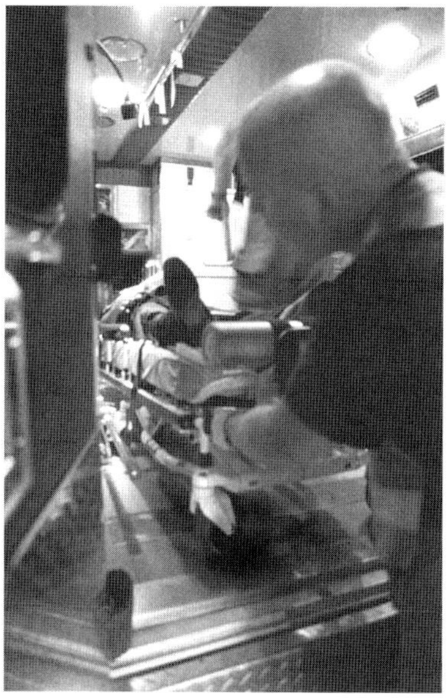

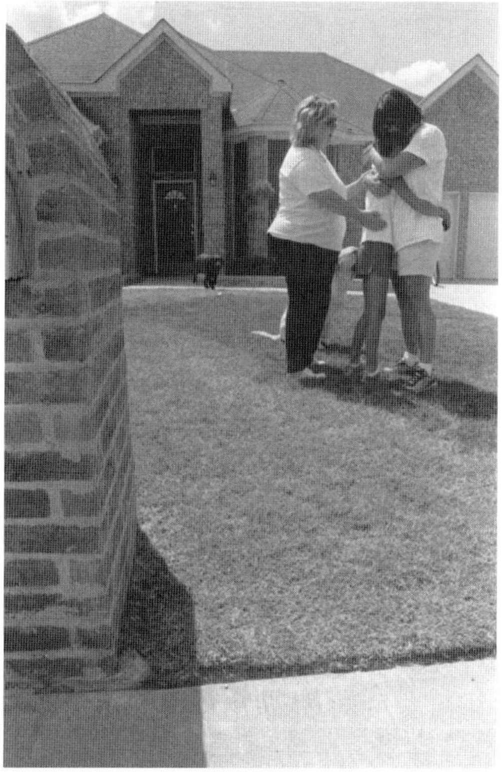

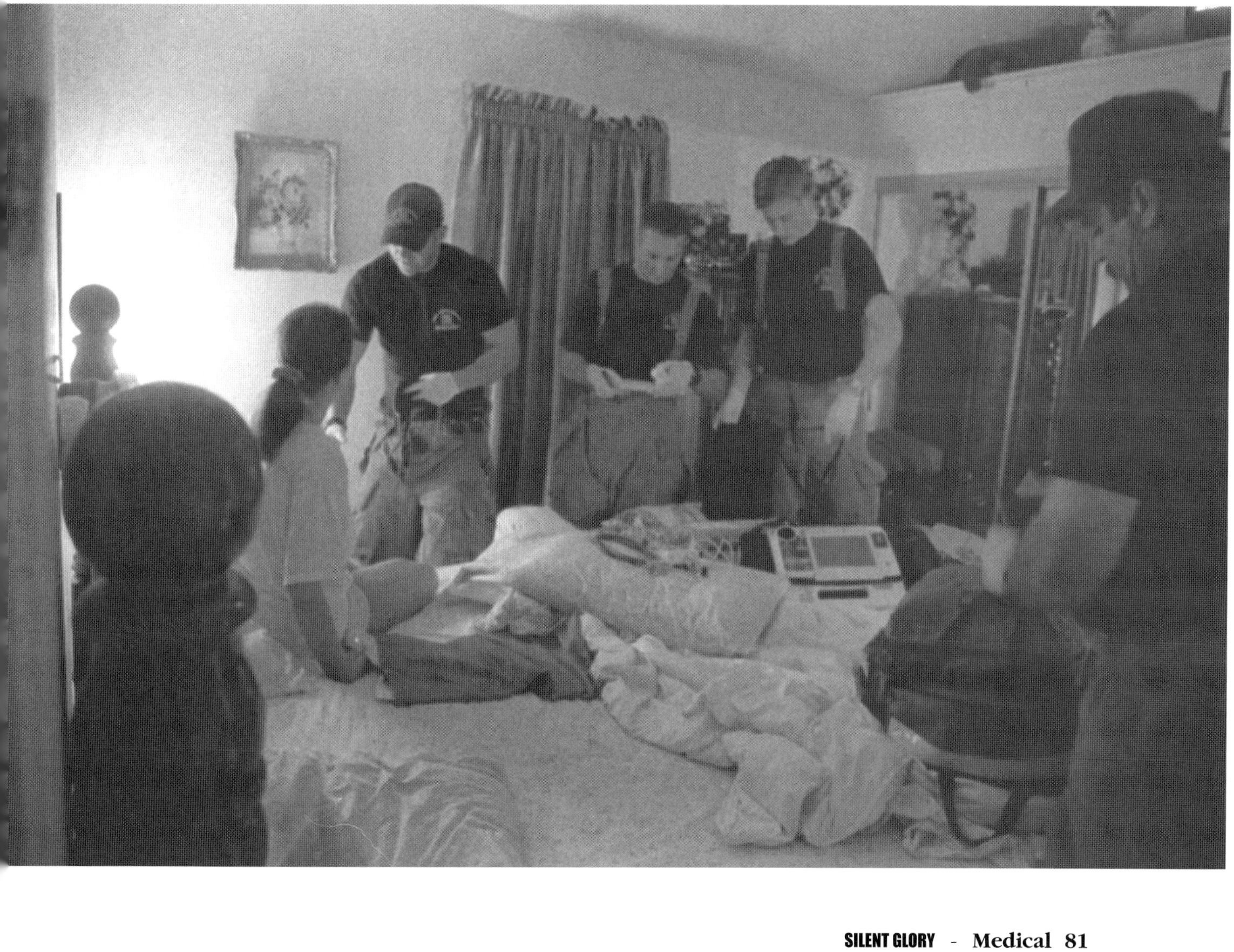

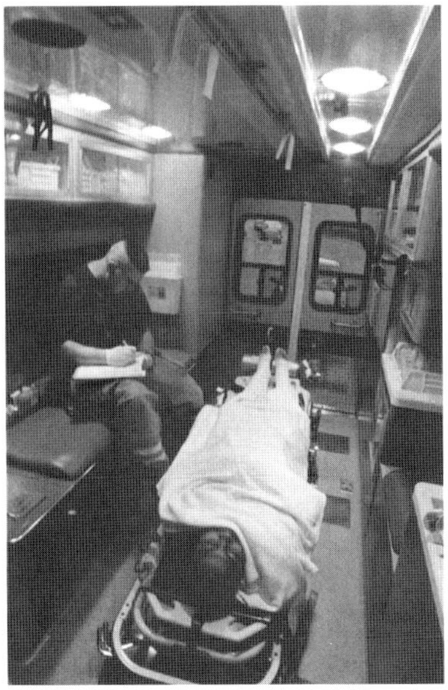

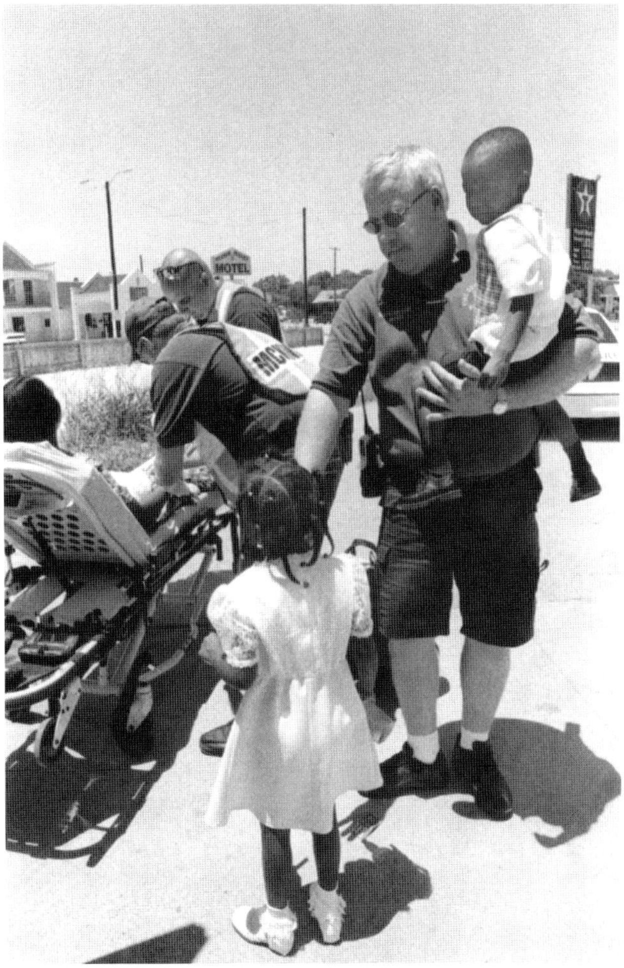
MOTEL

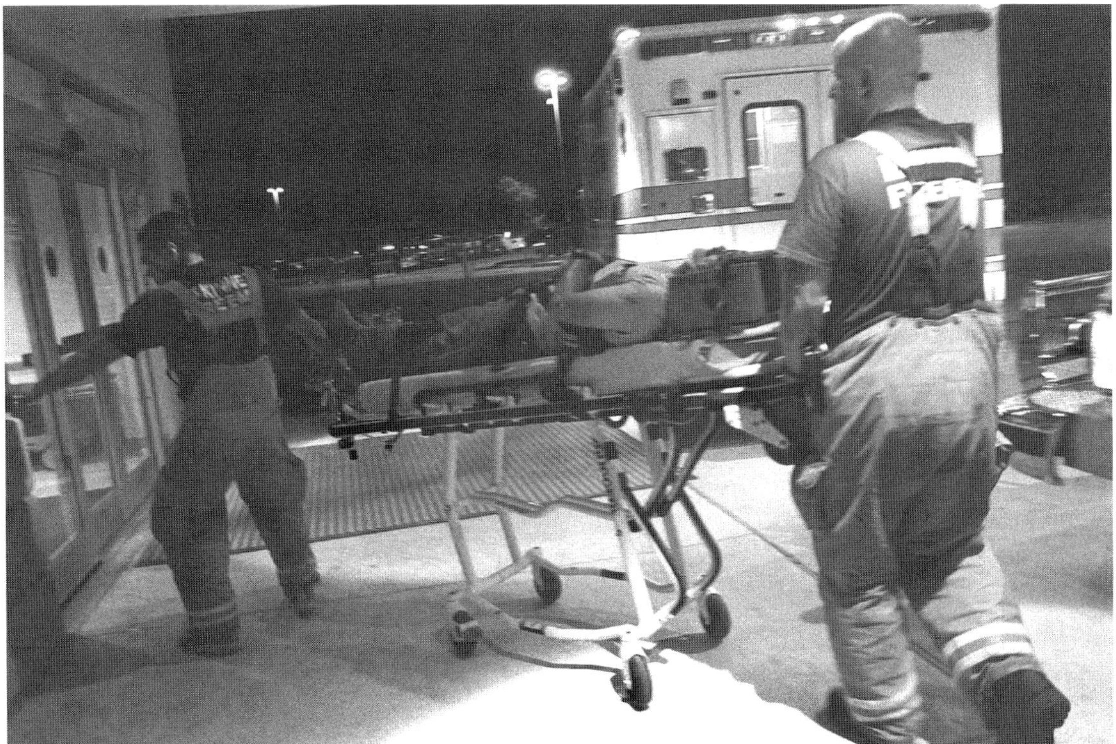

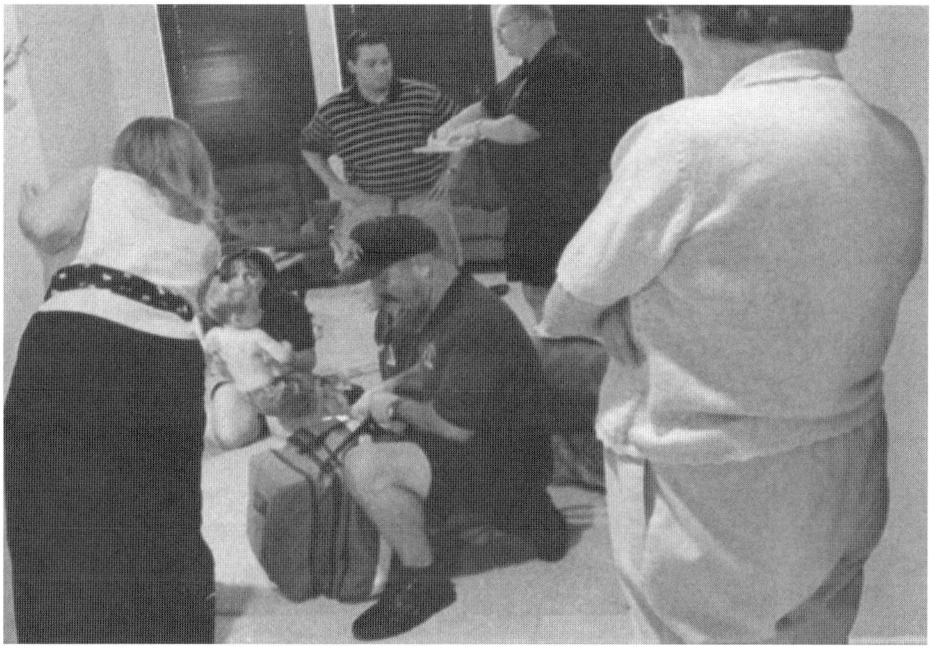

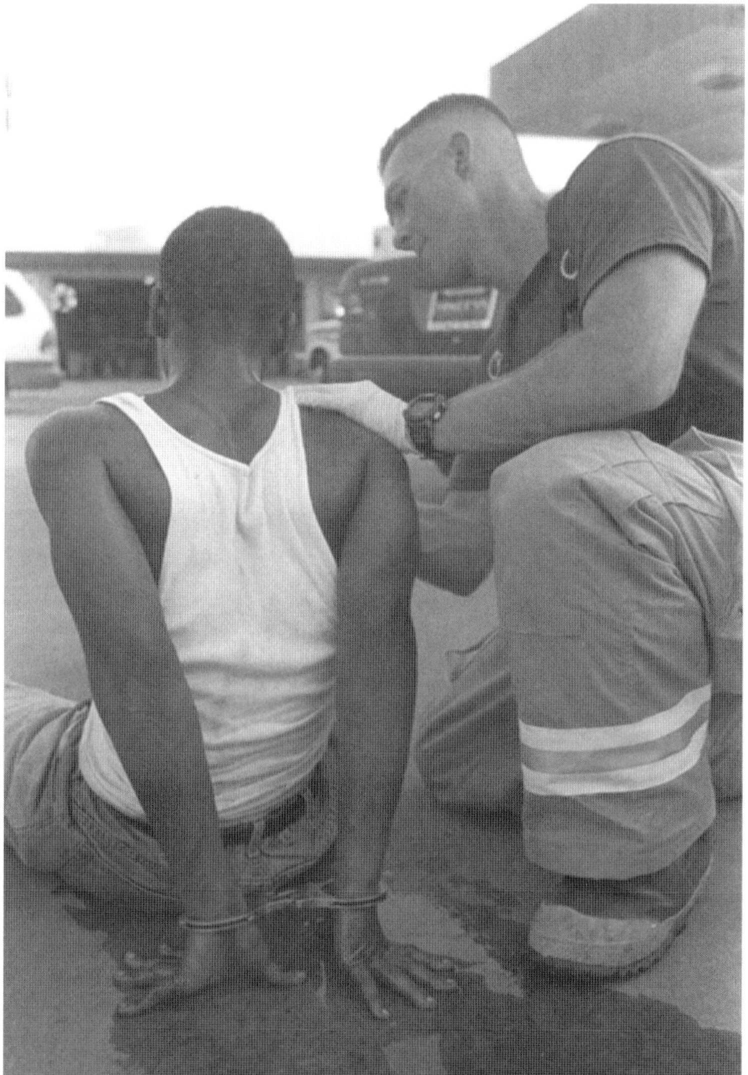

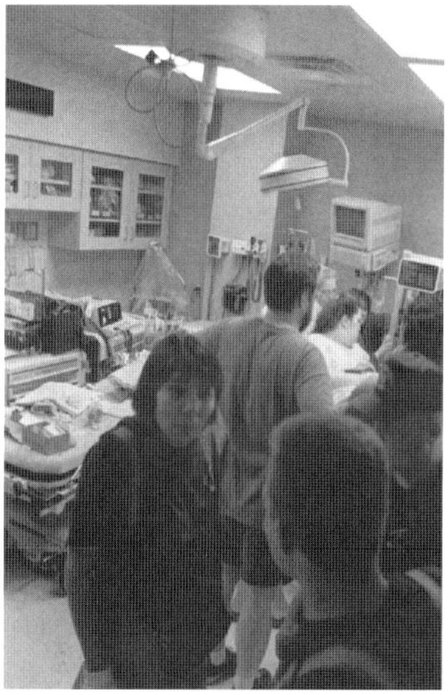

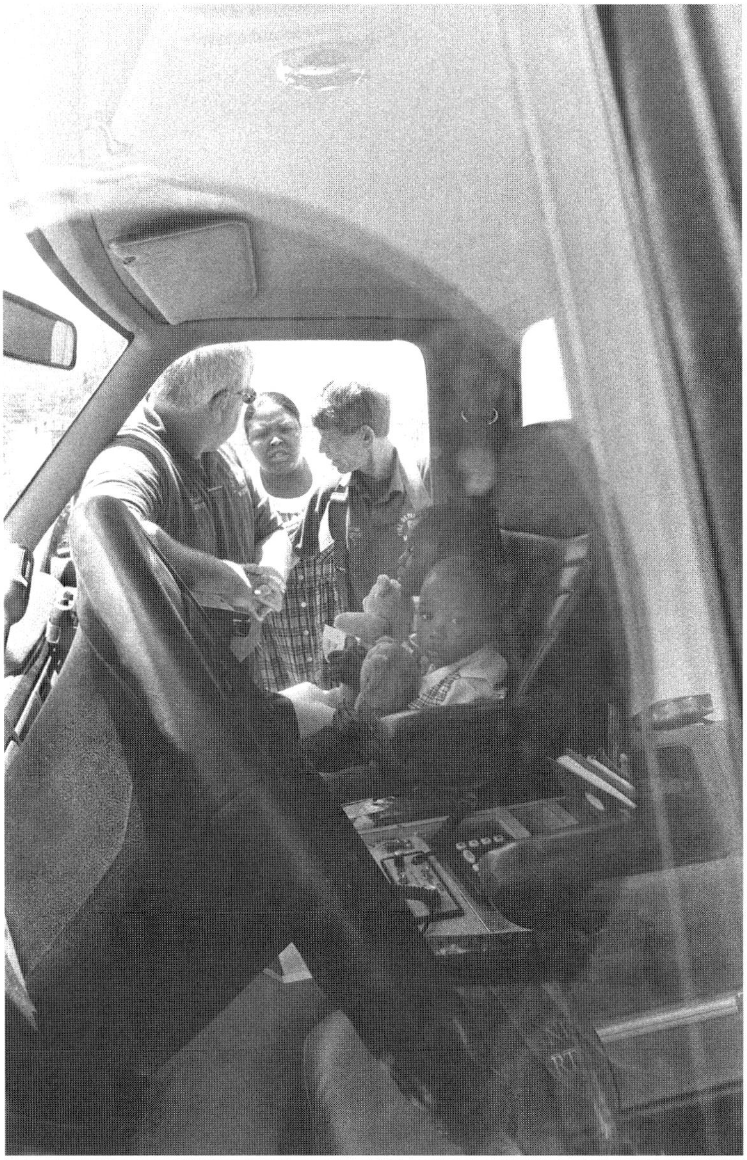

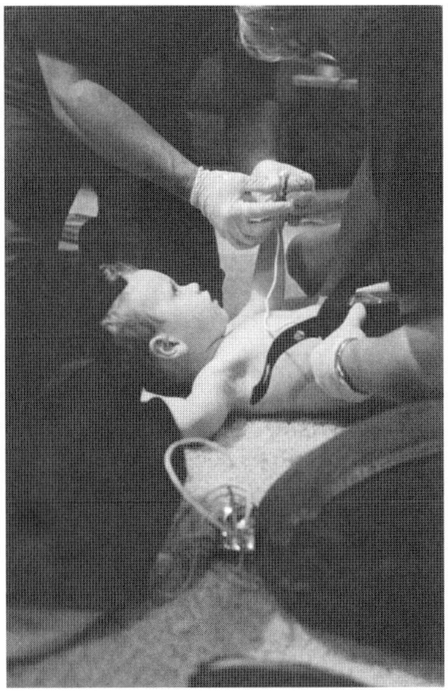

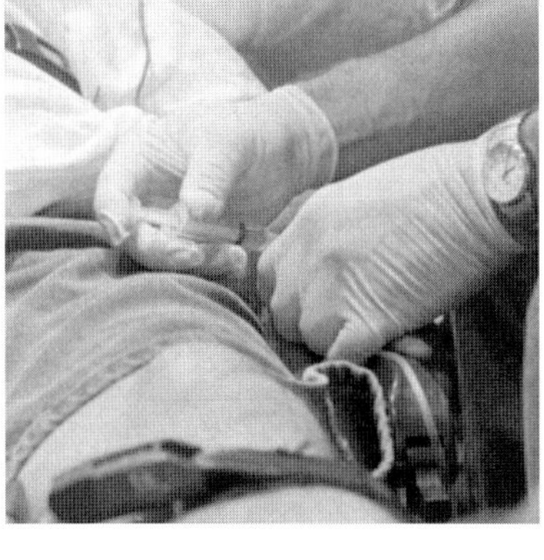

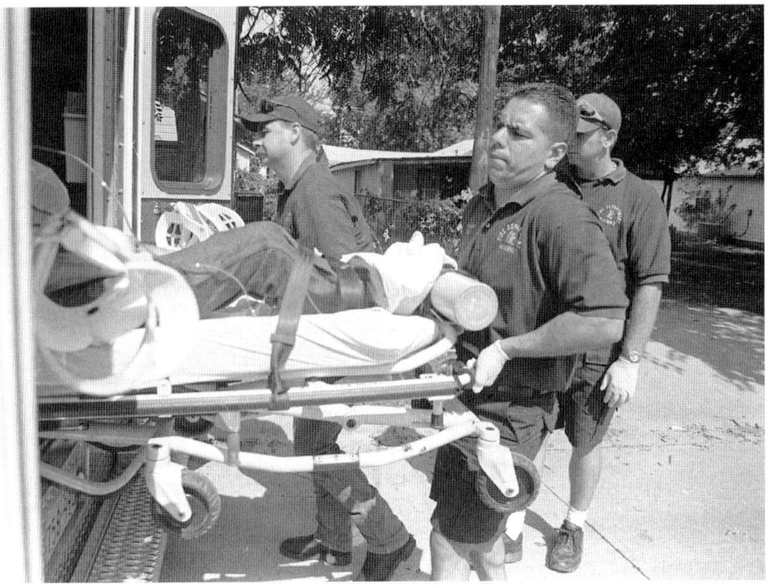

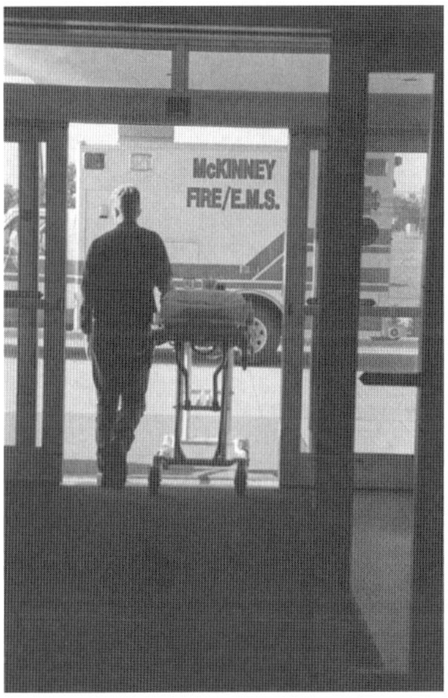
McKINNEY
FIRE/E.M.S.

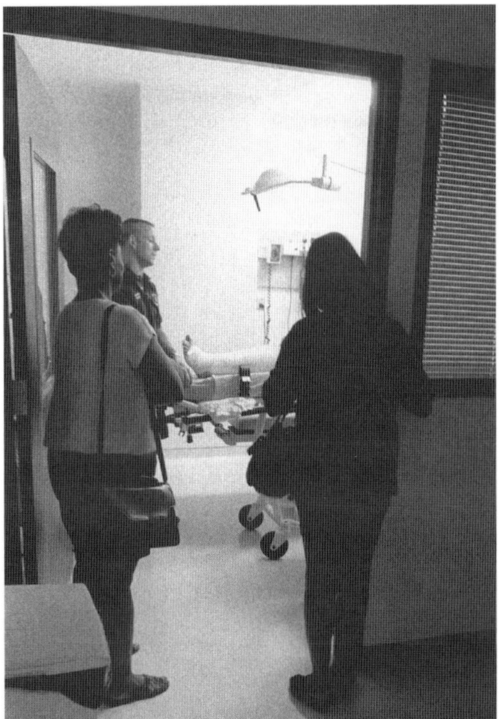

# training

Ever drive by a firehouse and wonder what's going on inside? Think they're playing cards or watching TV and wishing you had such leisure time on your job? Think again.

Probability is they are either studying the latest fire fighting techniques or training on their new mobile medical monitor. If they're out, they may be doing their "CE's" (continuing education requirements) at the local hospital or fire training center. Study, study, train, train, practice, practice, it is not a sometime thing... it is an all-time requirement from rookie to Chief.

Often, the training is physical, sometimes it is very technical. Sometimes it's quite elementary; like instantly knowing the best route to a certain address when the call comes in for help in your town on your street at your house number. They know the fastest way to every home, on every street, by heart. And when they arrive, they know exactly what to do.

Basic, but essential.

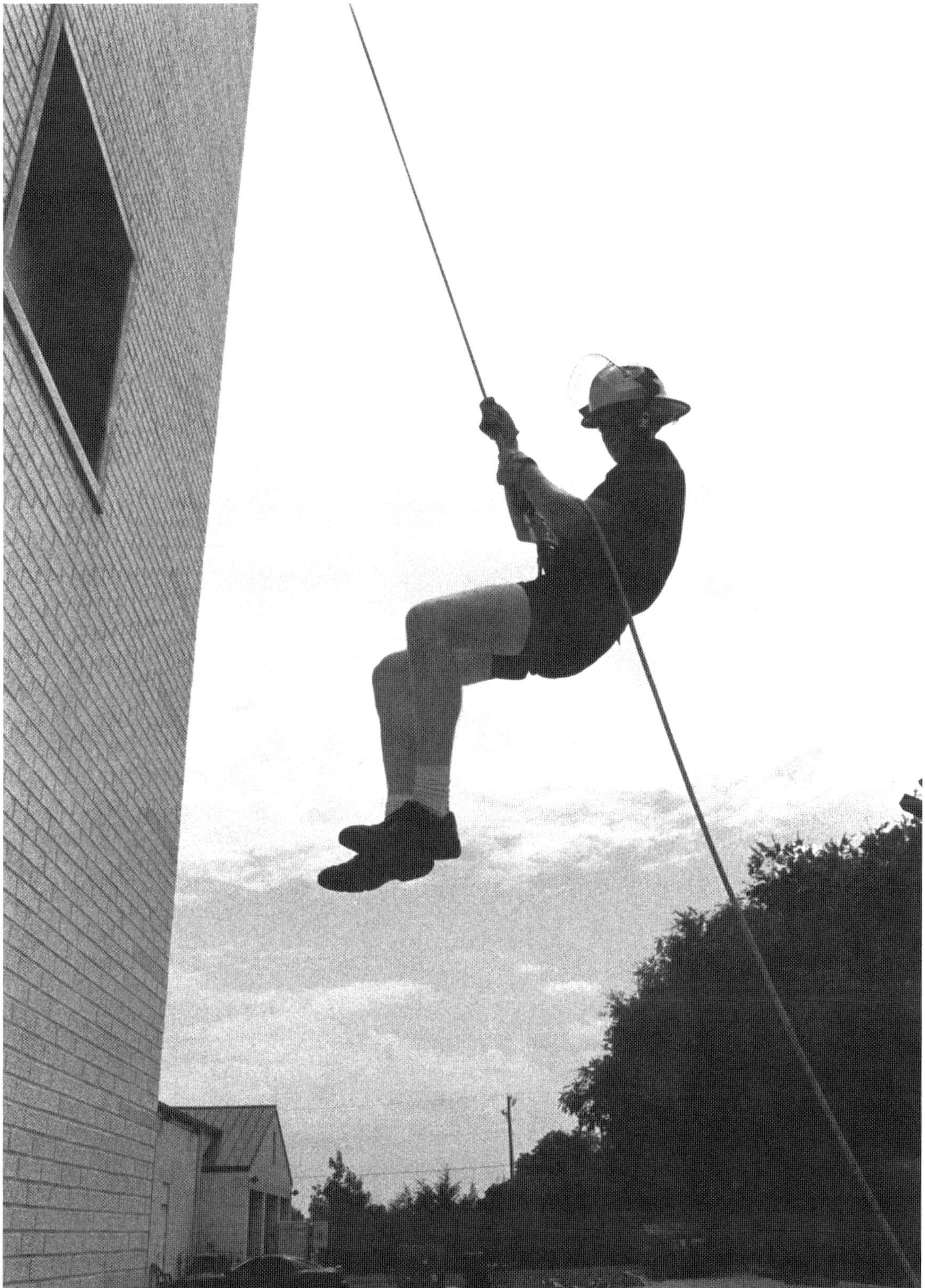

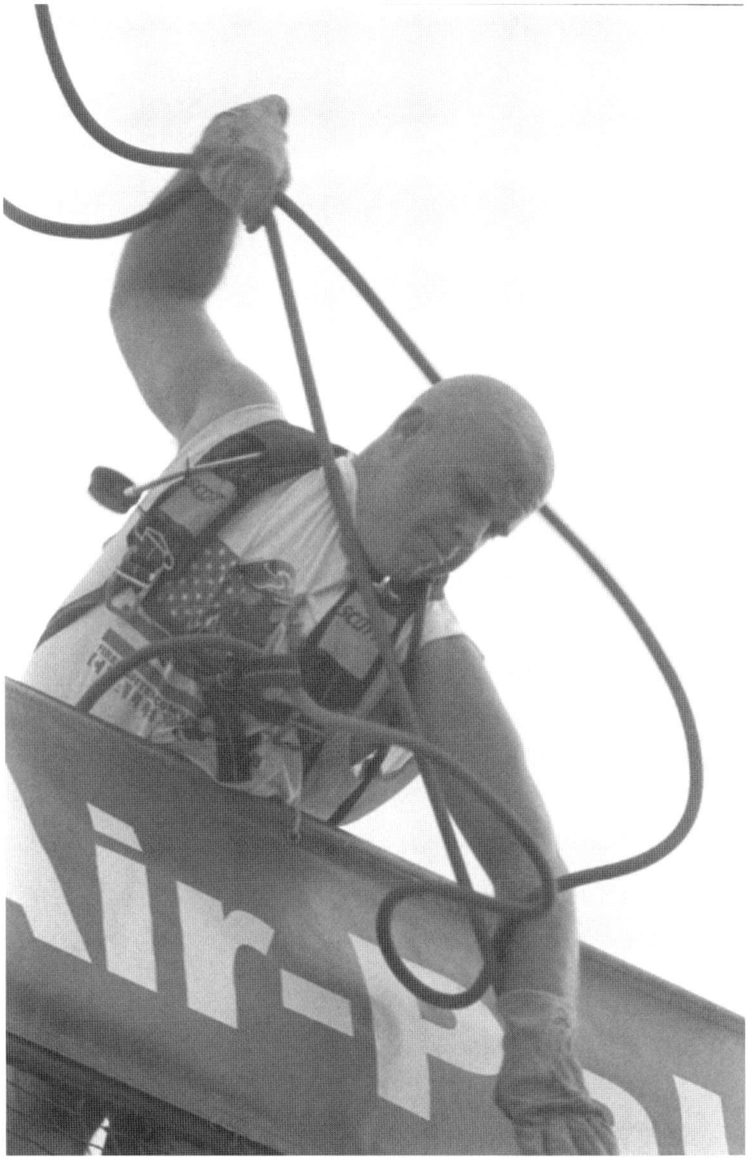
Air-P

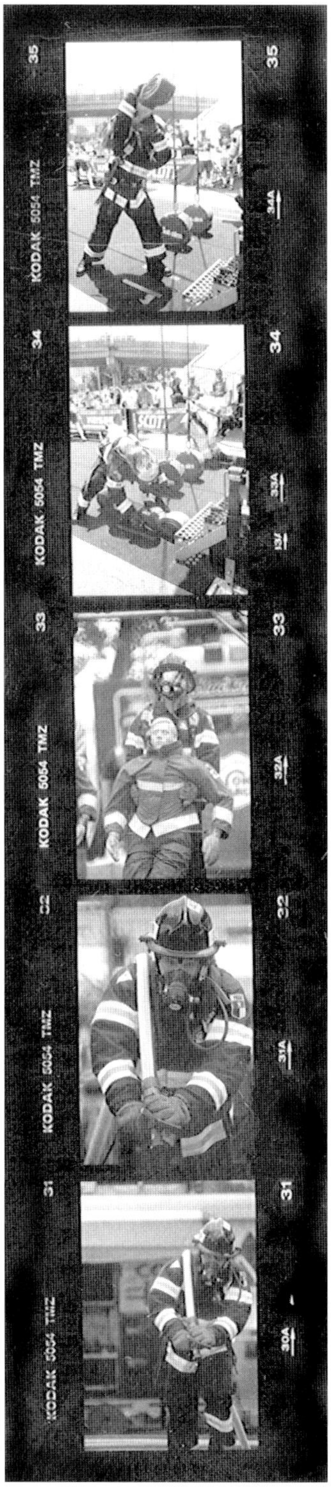
KODAK 5054 TMZ

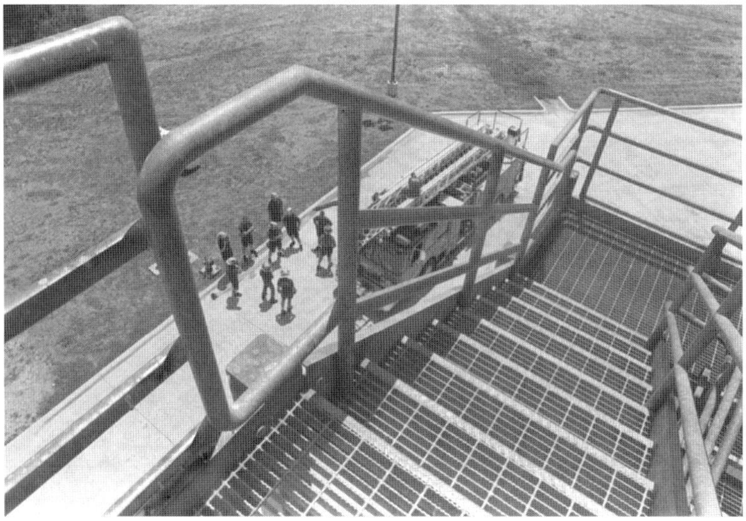

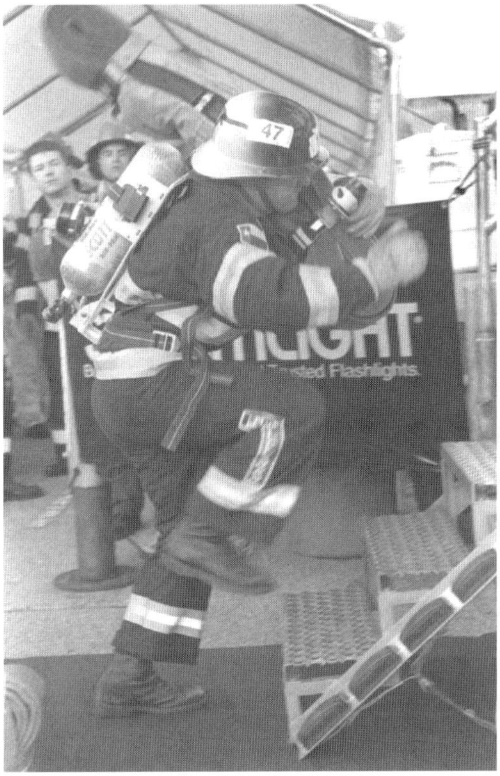
47

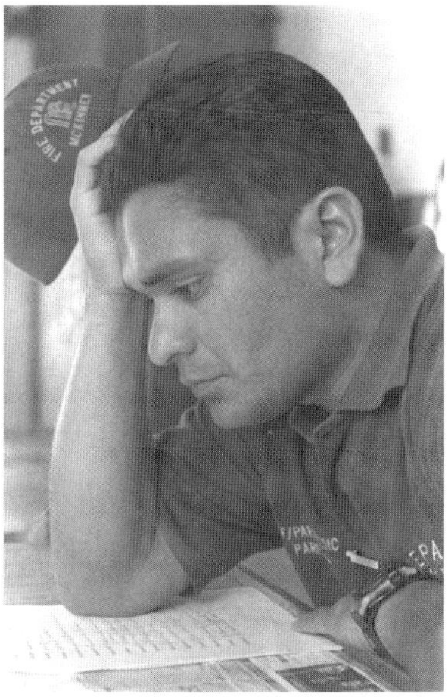

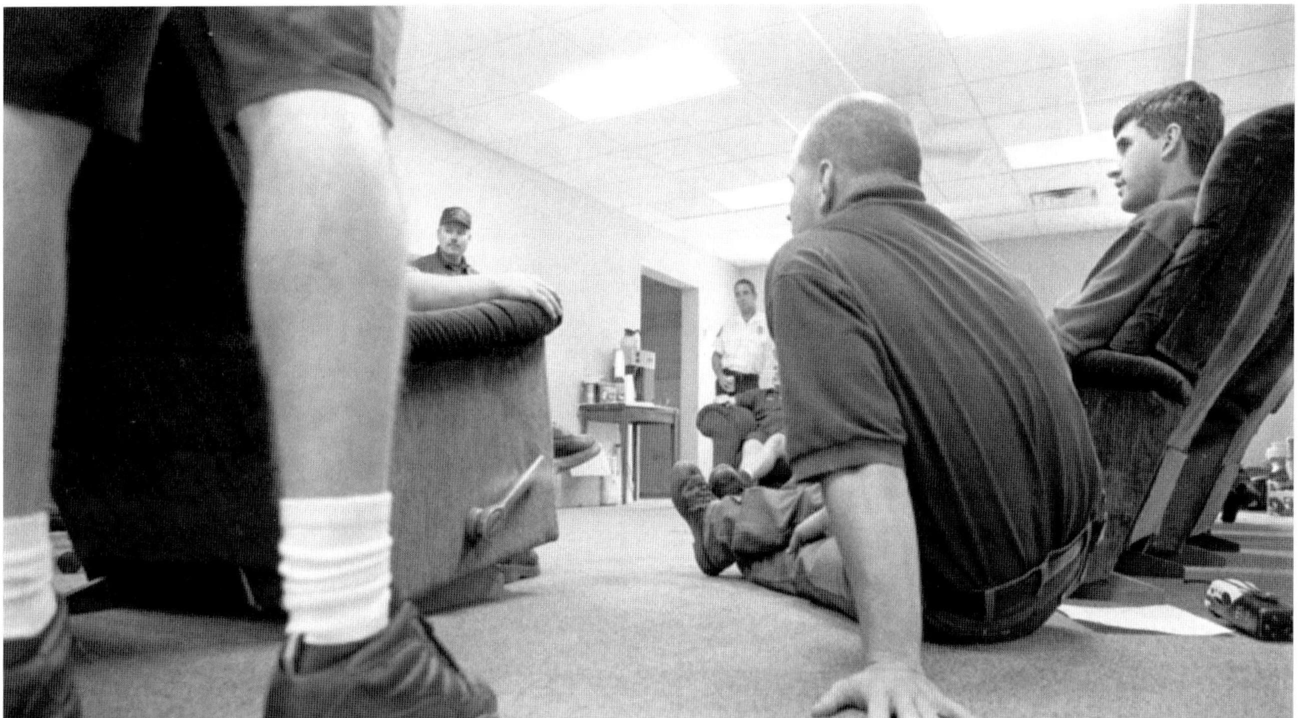

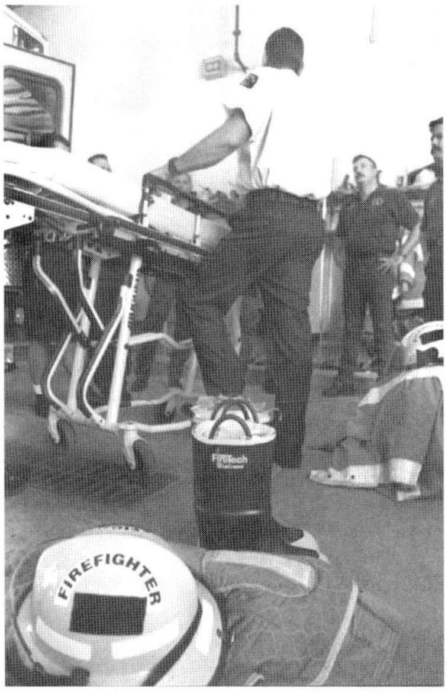
FIREFIGHTER

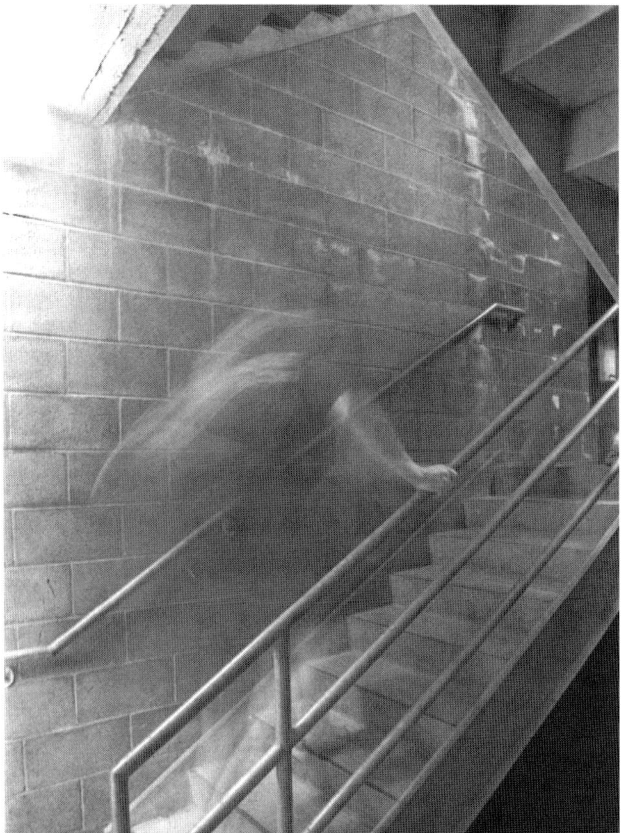

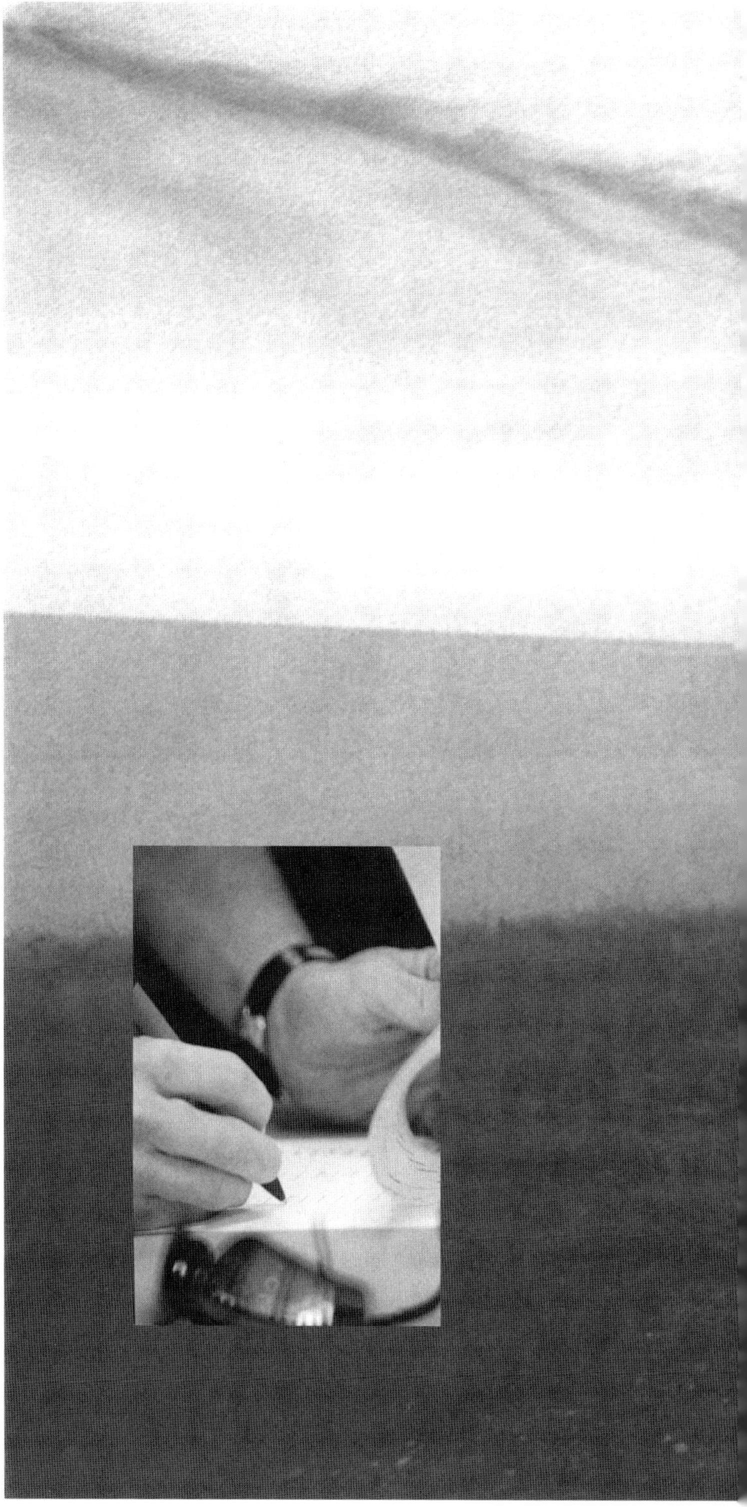

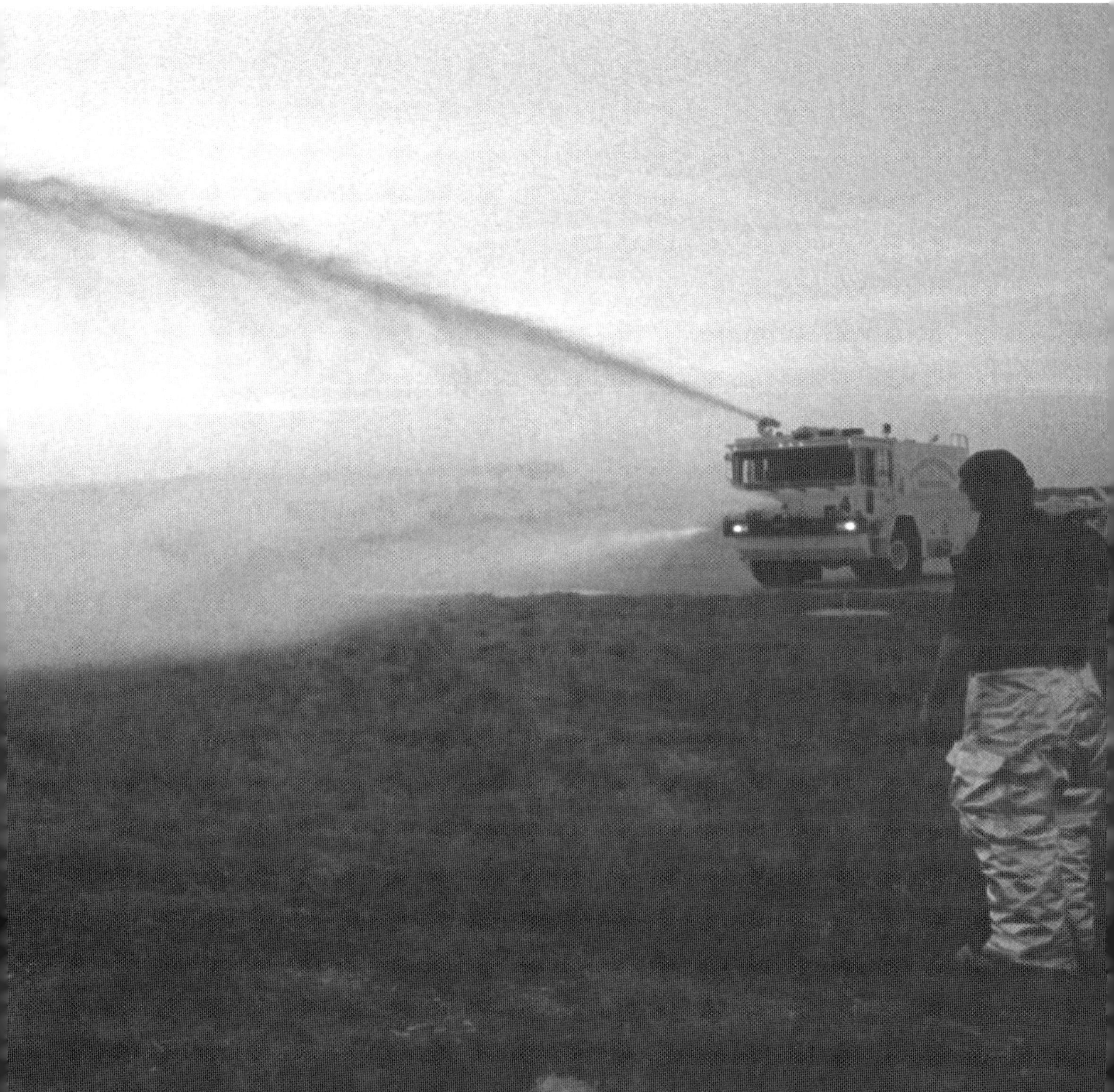

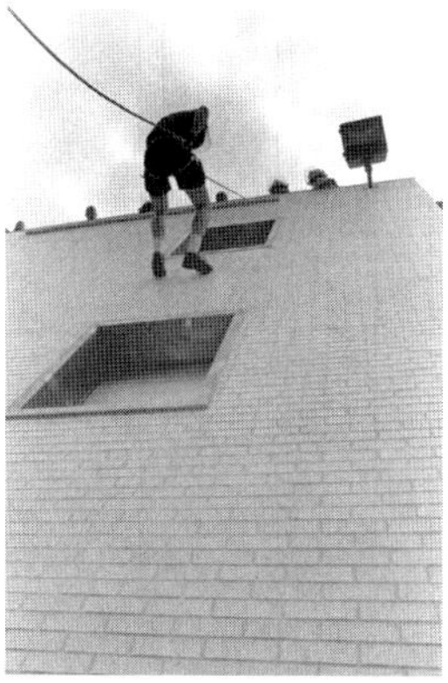
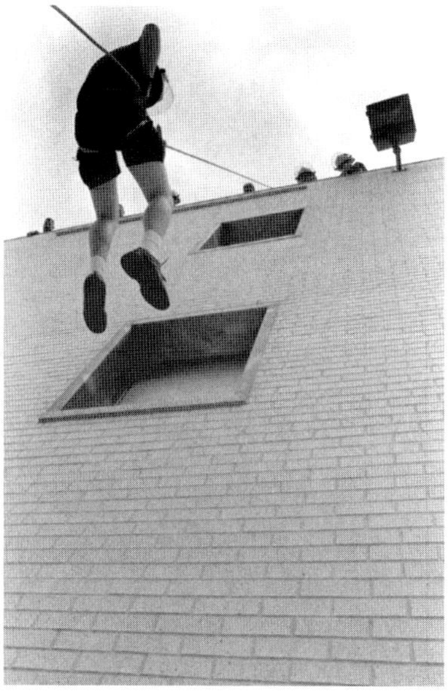
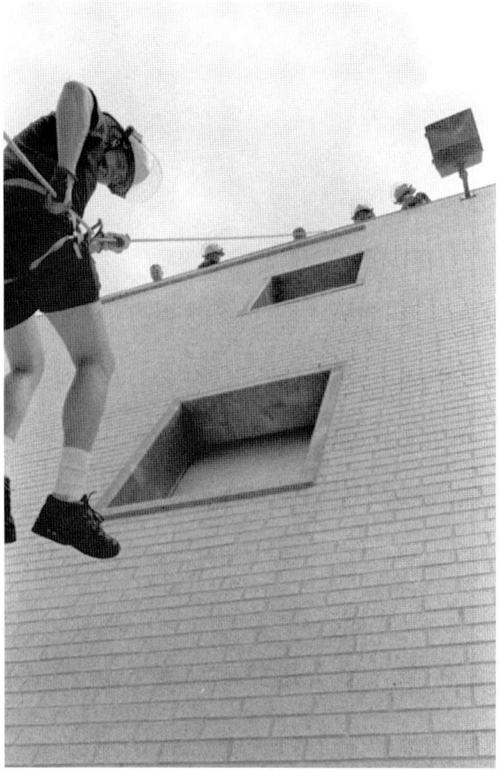

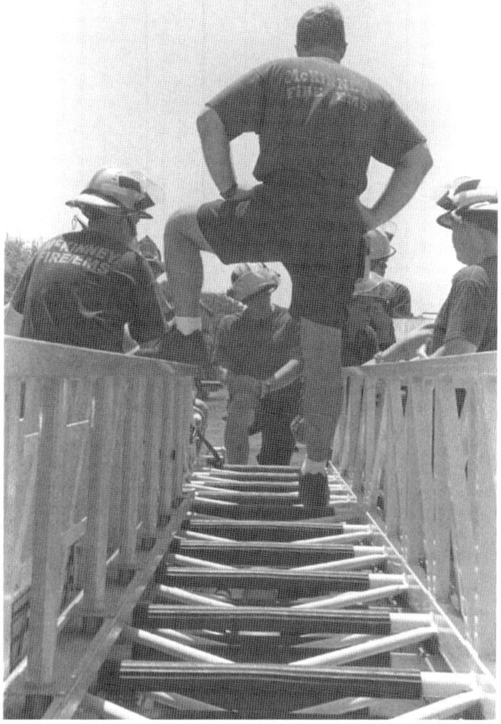

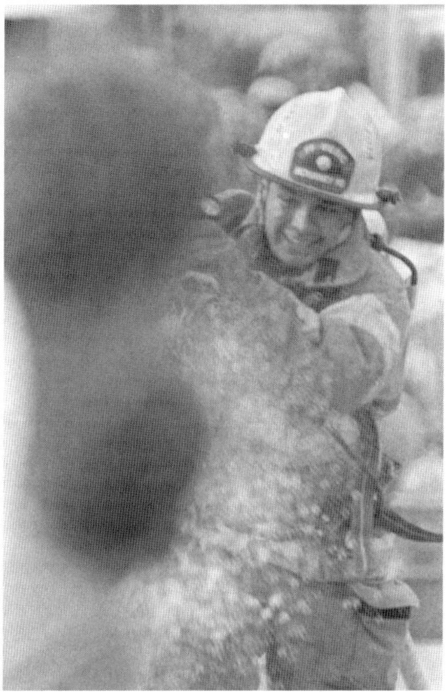

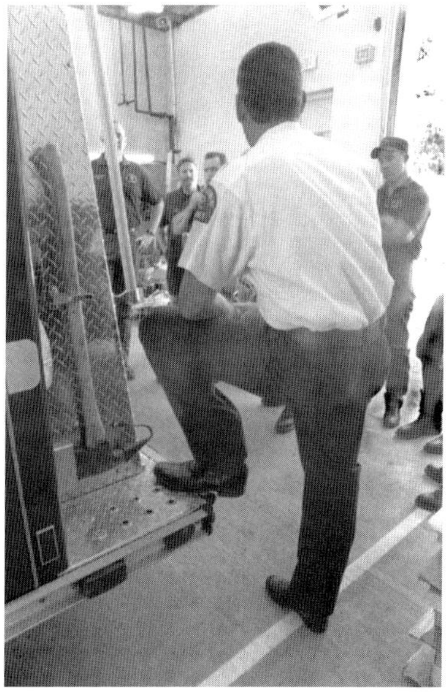

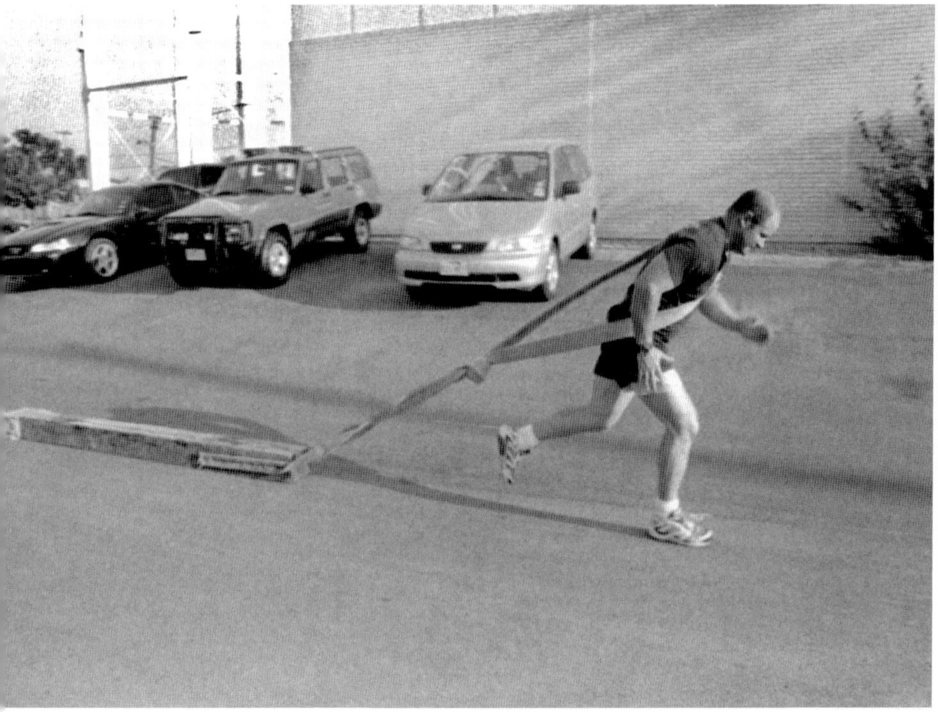

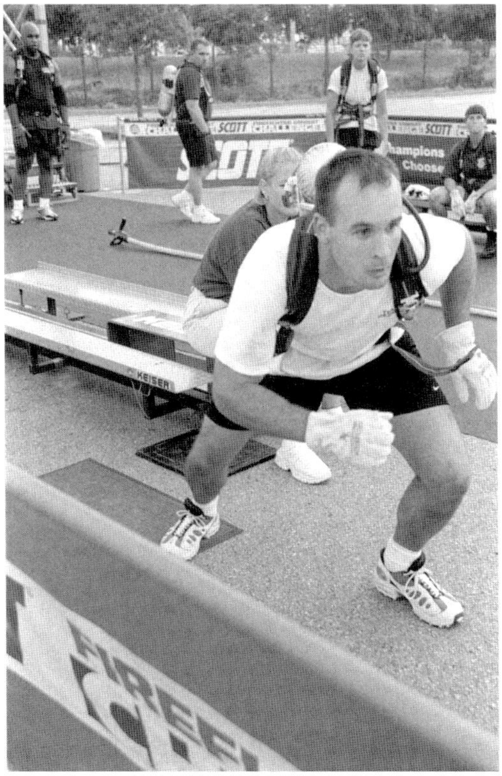
SCOTT
KEISER

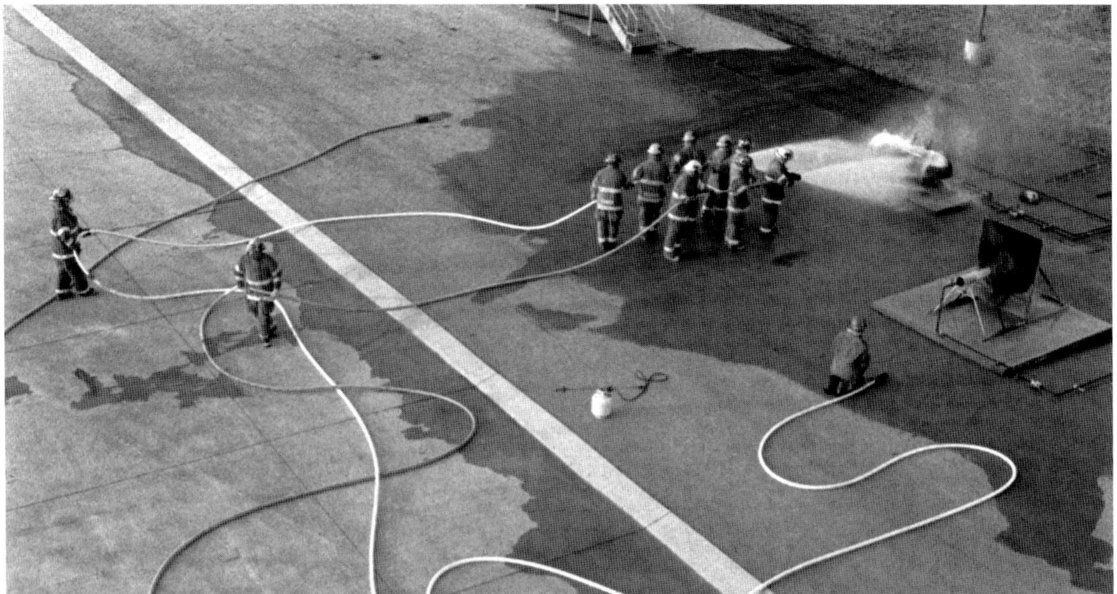

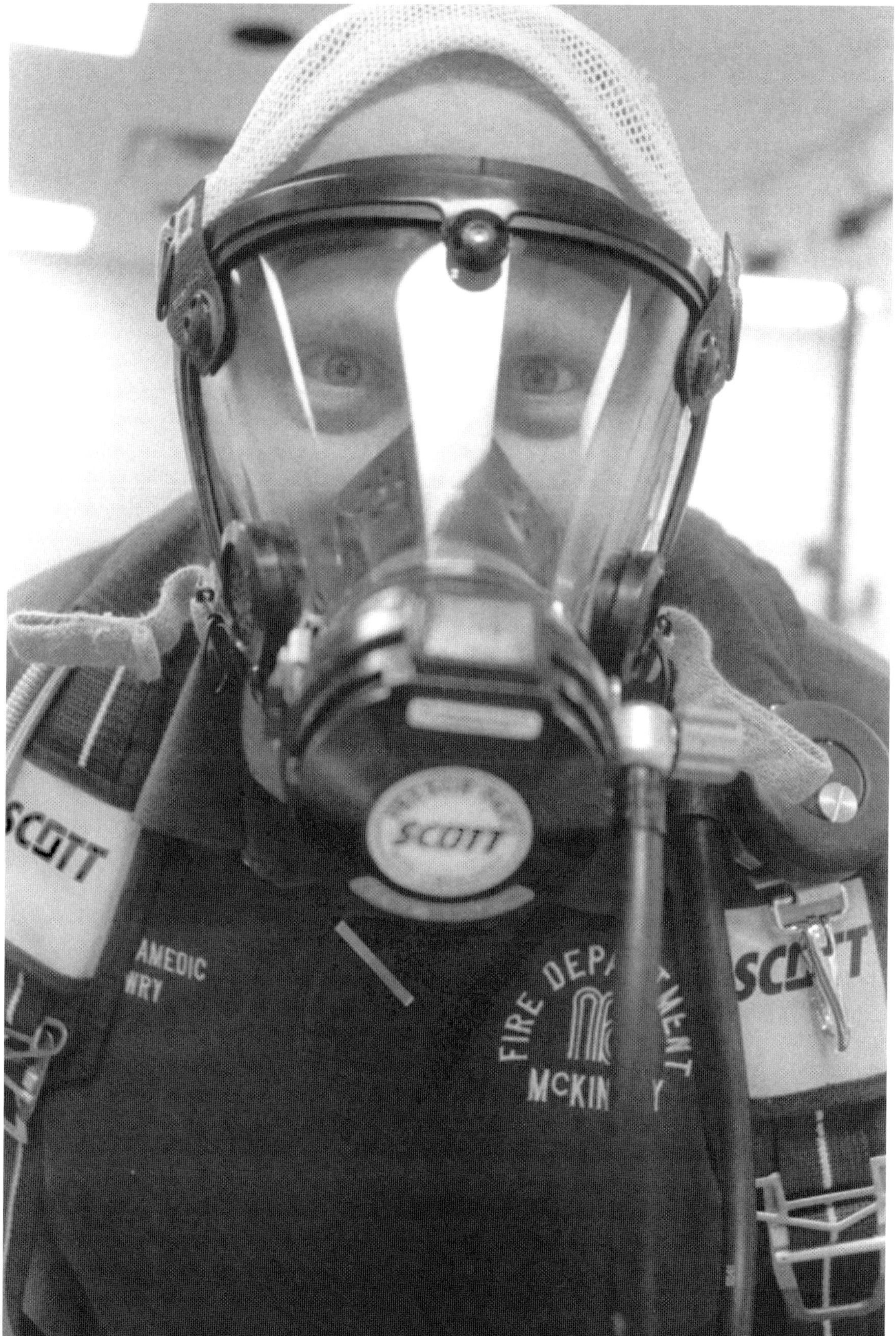
SCOTT
SCOTT

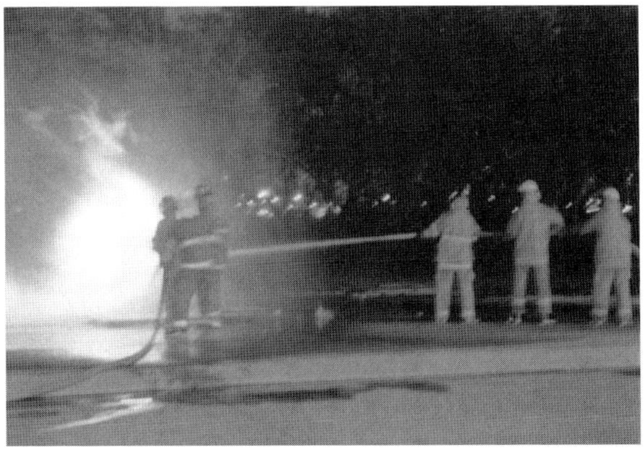

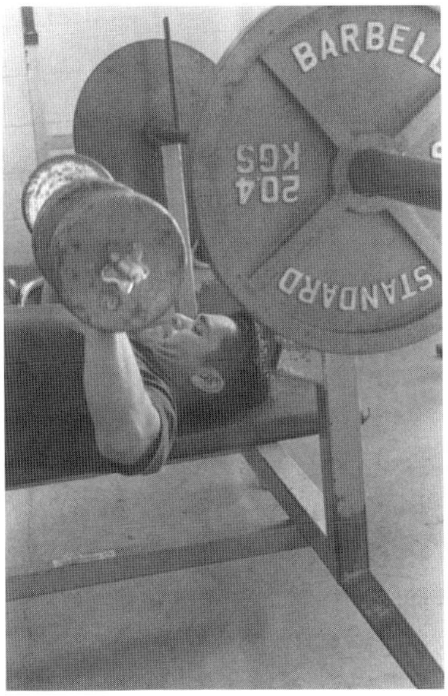
STANDARD

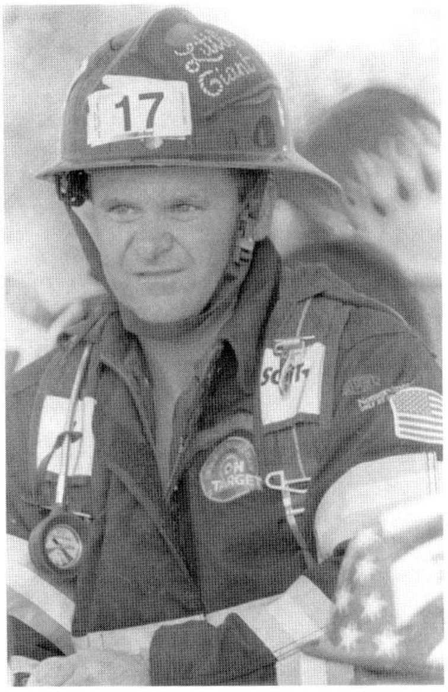
17

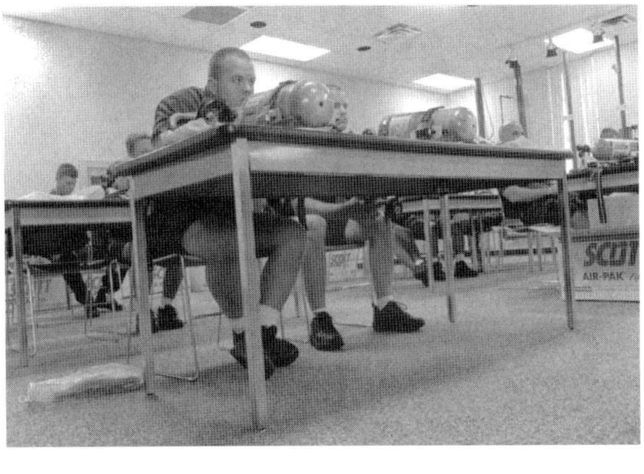
AIR-PAK

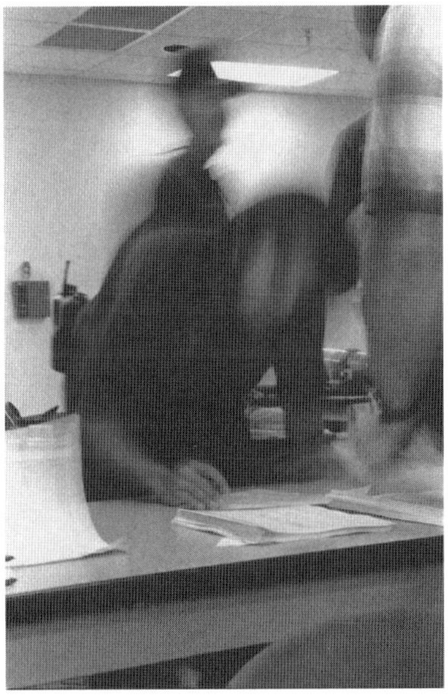
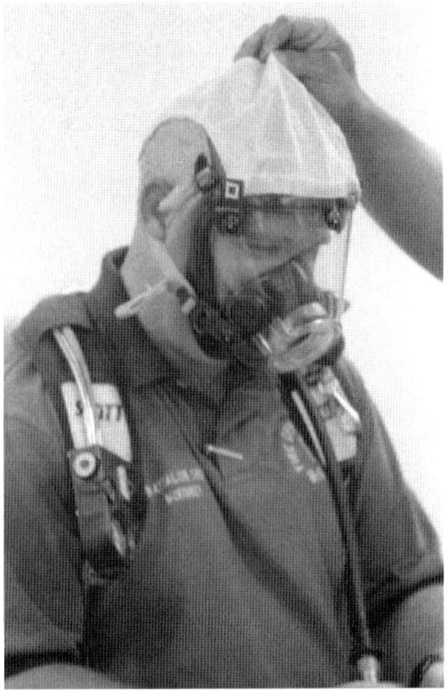
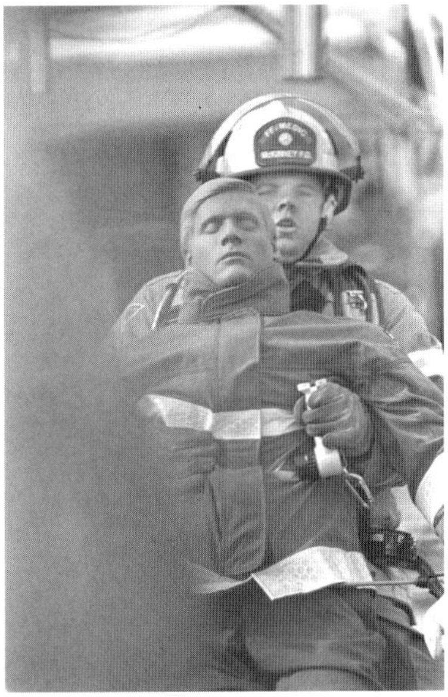
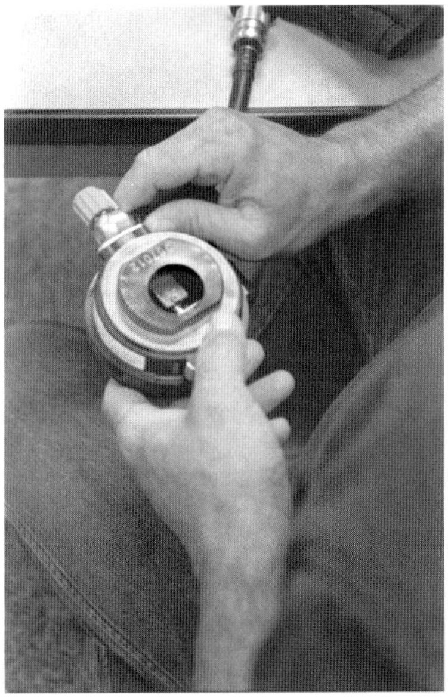

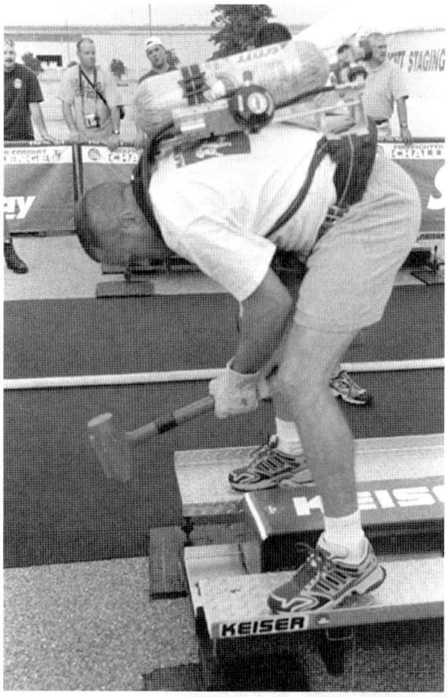
KEISER

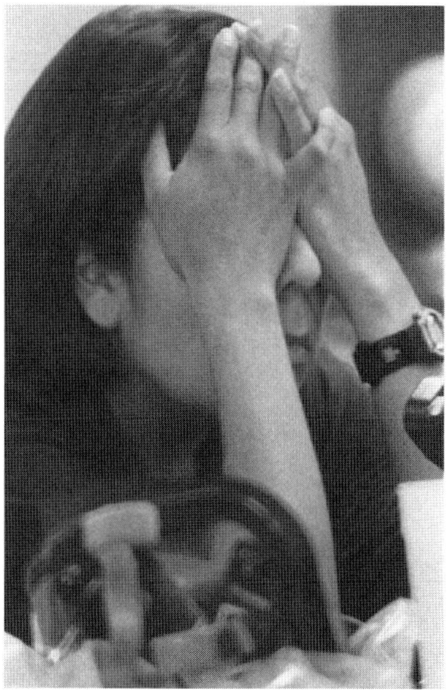

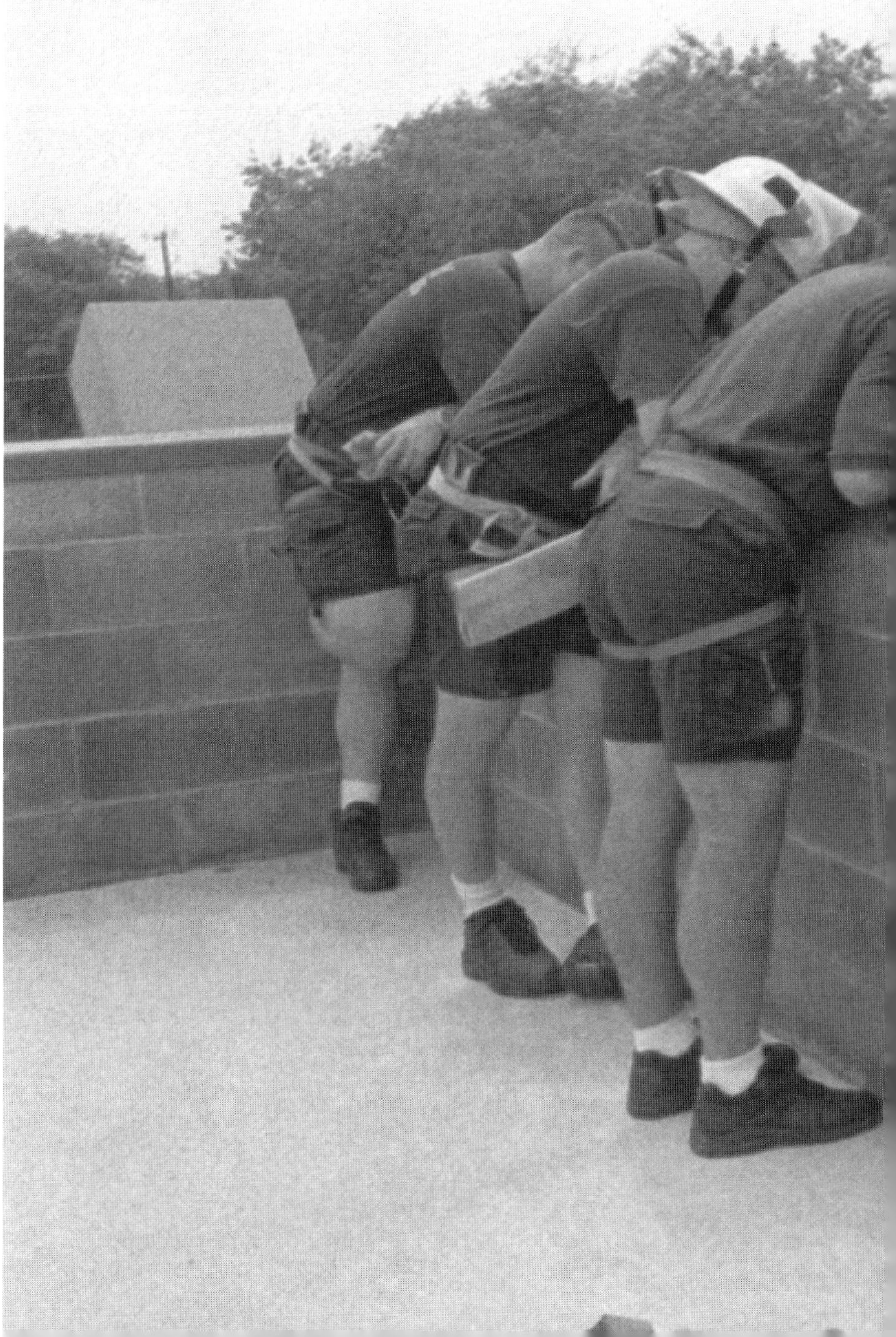

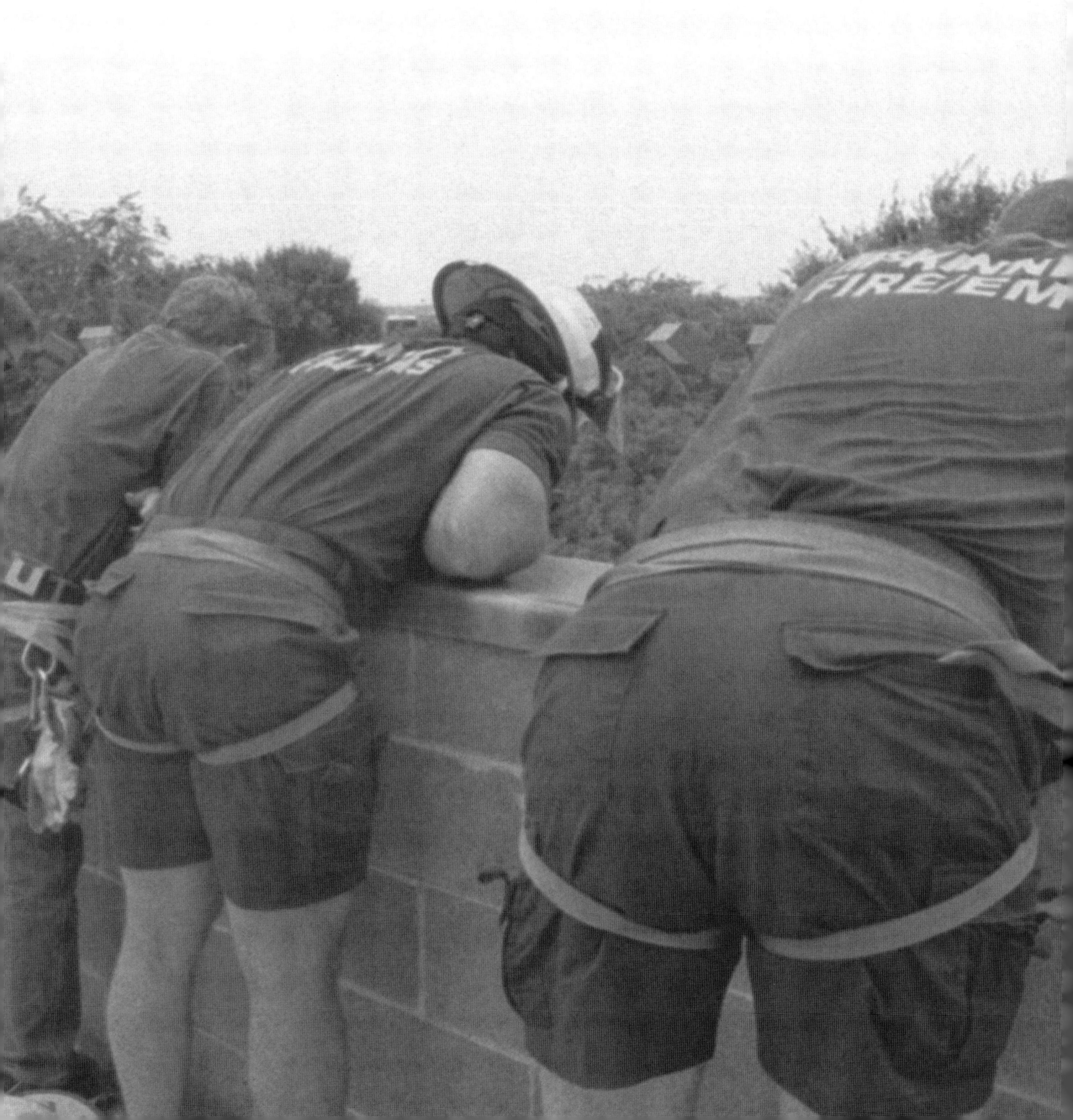

# equipment

The equipment used by today's Firefighters range from a simple axe, to a complex 100' ladder truck, to the "jaws of life", to the most modern mobile medical devices that defy the imagination.

But each item is virtually useless unless it is available, maintained and working, to say nothing of the operator's training. Each piece used by Firefighters is a precious and irreplaceable element of their work. Every Firefighter treasures each tool and device made available to them. They guard it and maintain it with their life so that yours is protected by it.

Consider a Firefighters air tank and regulator. Now consider if **you** were a Firefighter, how important would it be that it is the best breathing support system available and in perfect working order? How important would it be if... **you** are the person trapped by fire and smoke the Firefighter is trying to rescue?

When the call goes out for a volunteer fire department donation or voter approval for a fire equipment bond issue, think of the possibility that your life, loved ones, home or business and the Firefighters' lives depend on the wish list items being in their hands when your desperate call for help comes in.

Think about it again.

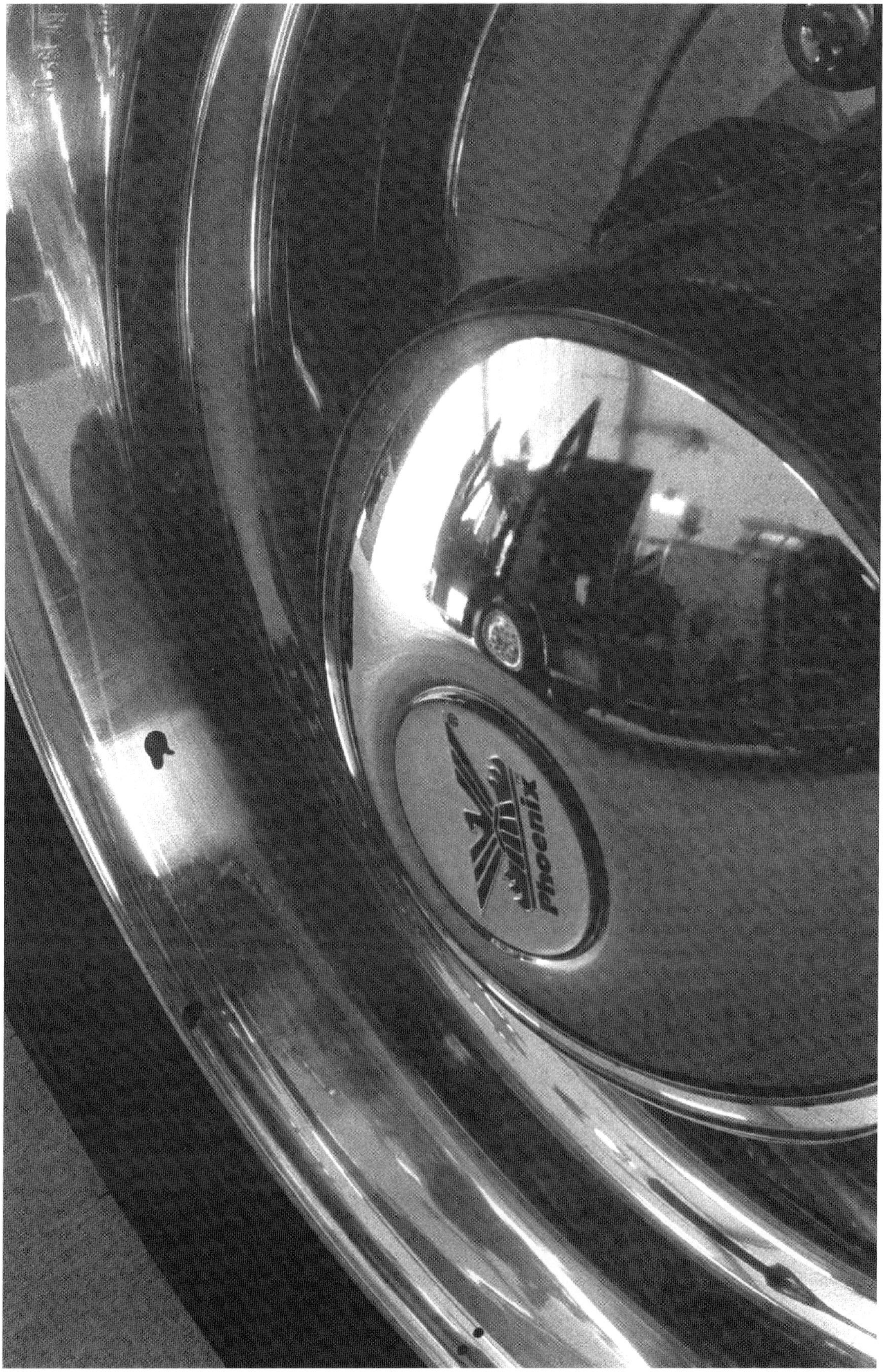
Phoenix

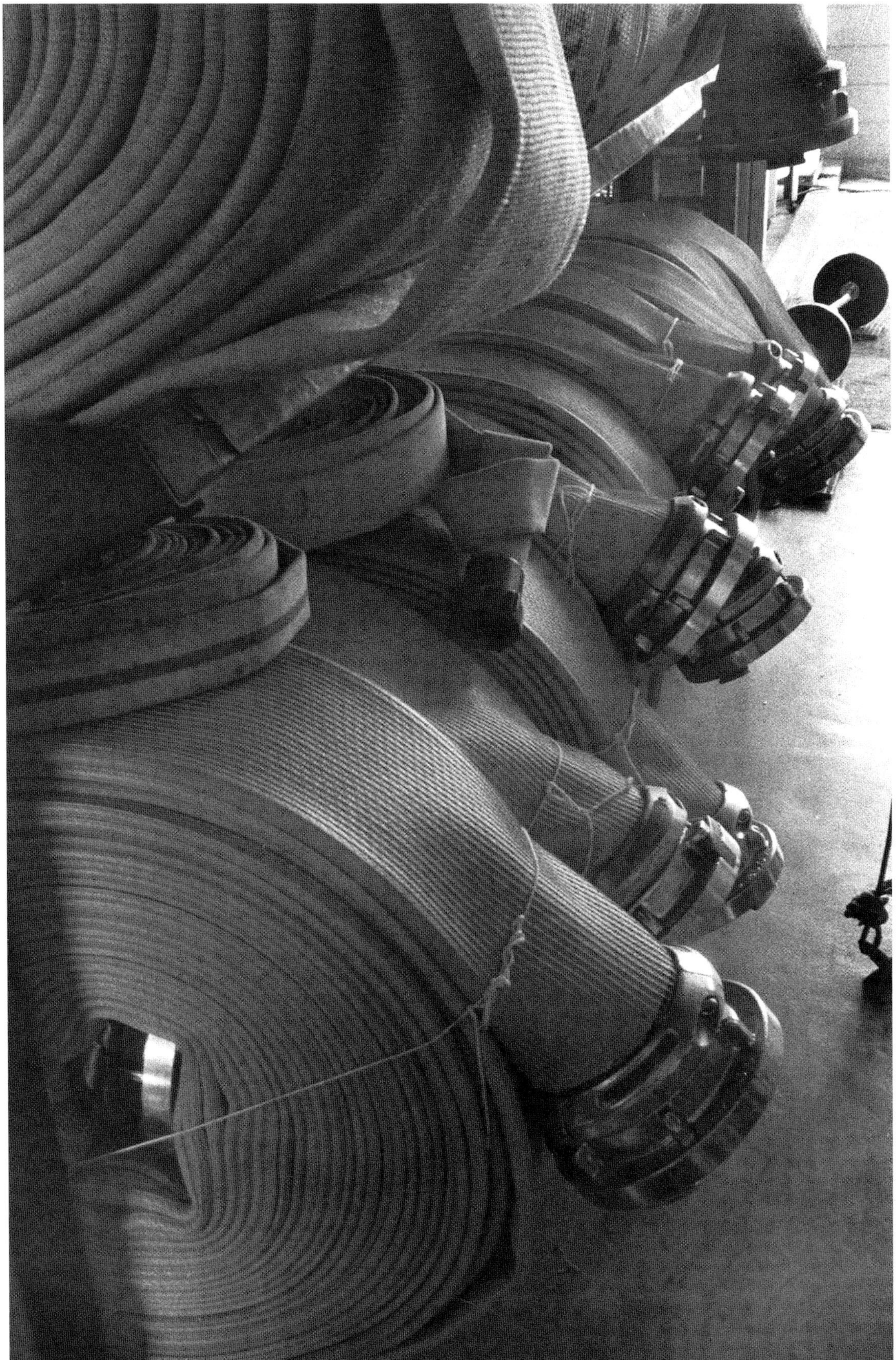

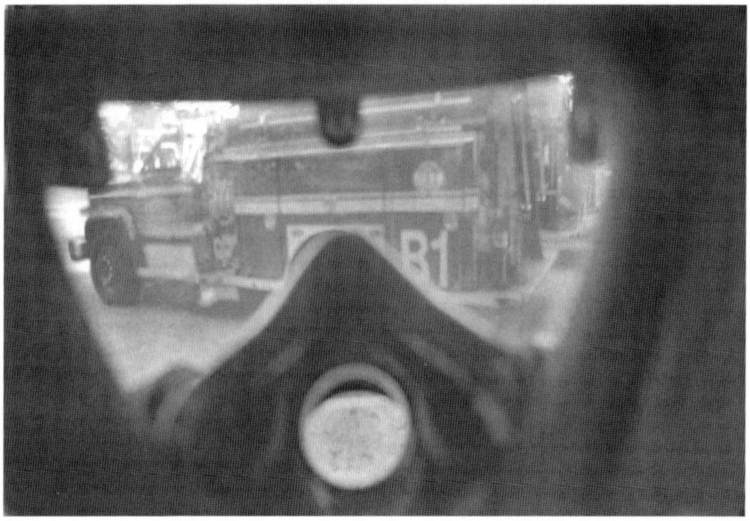

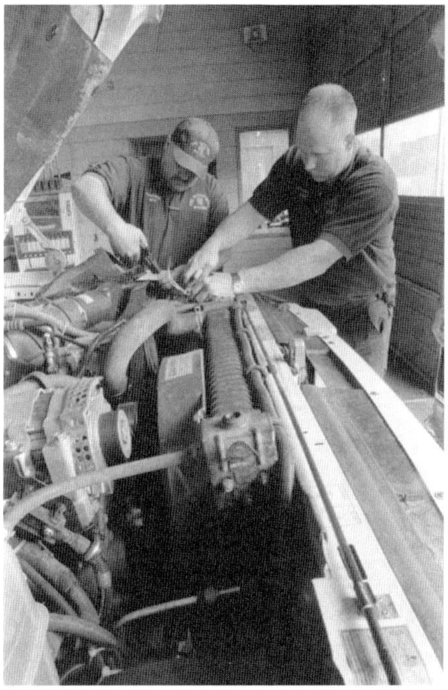

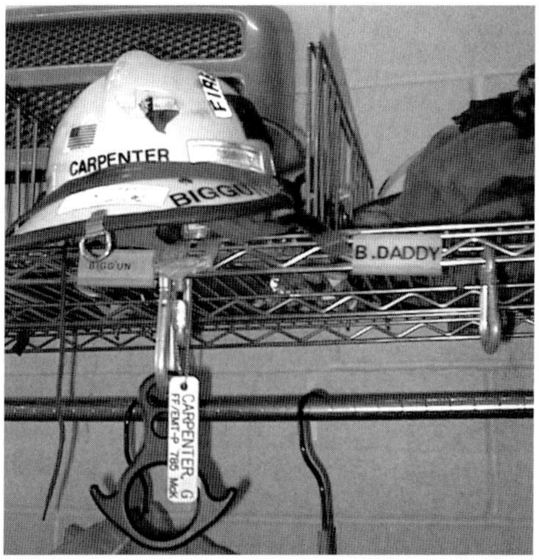
CARPENTER
B.DADDY
CARPENTER, G

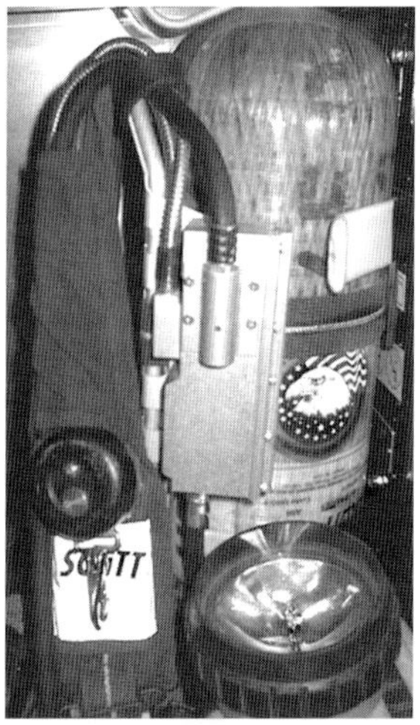
SCOTT

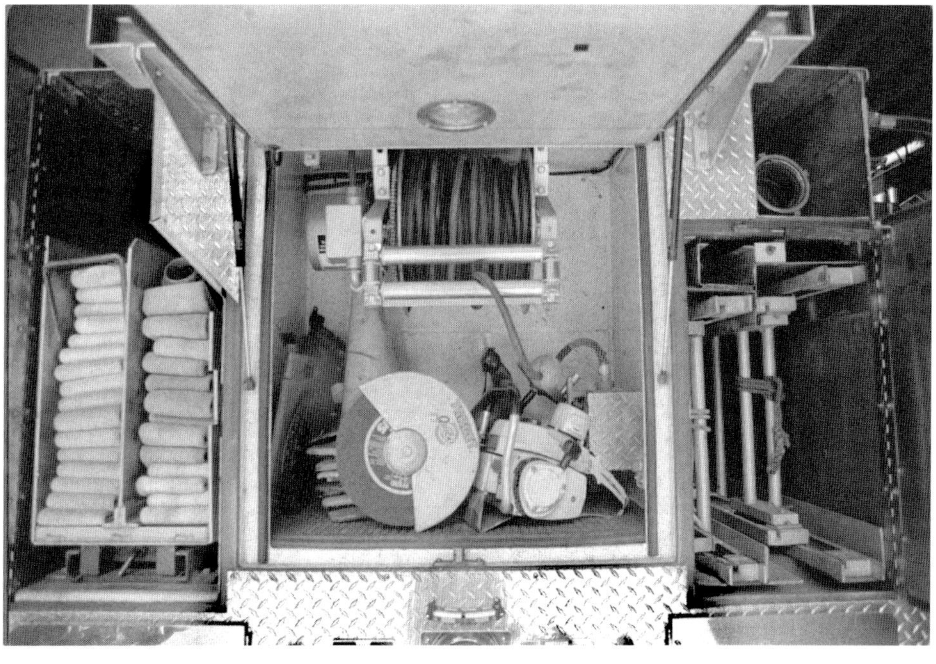

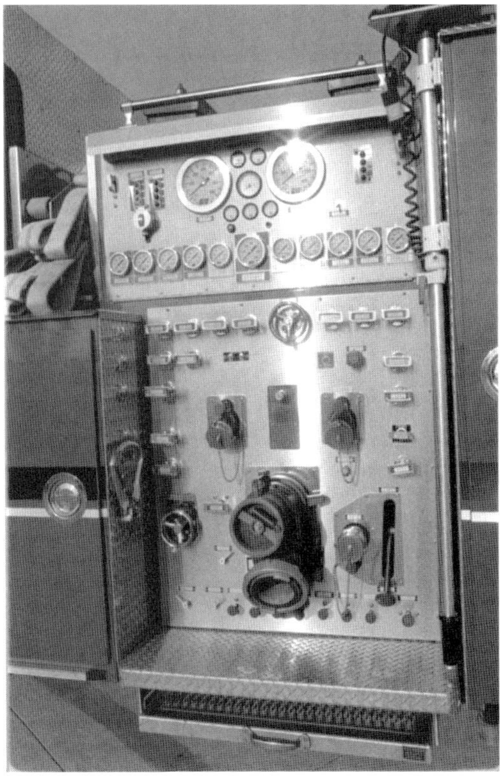

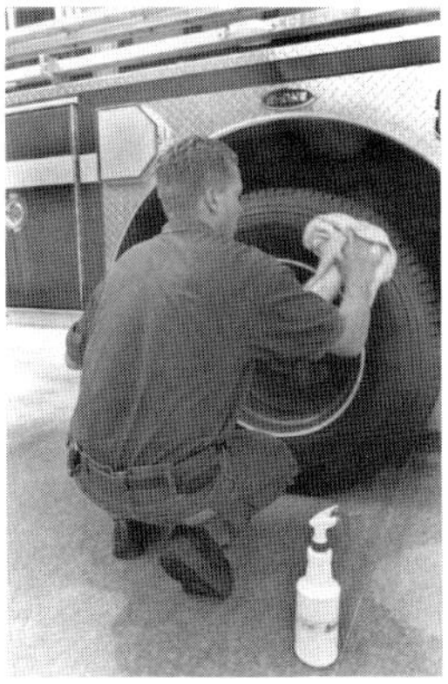

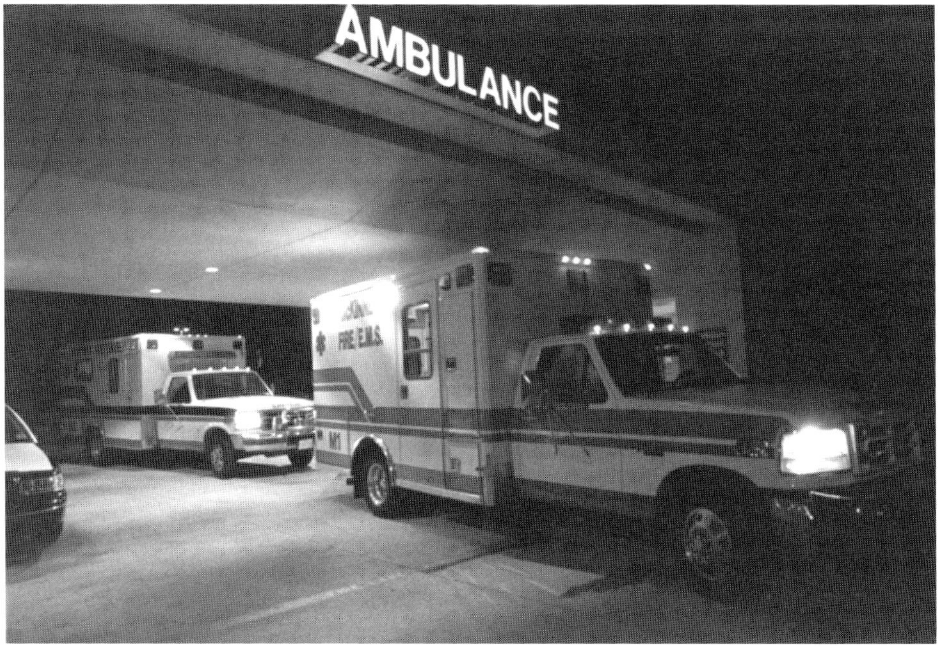
AMBULANCE
FIRE/E.M.S.
M1

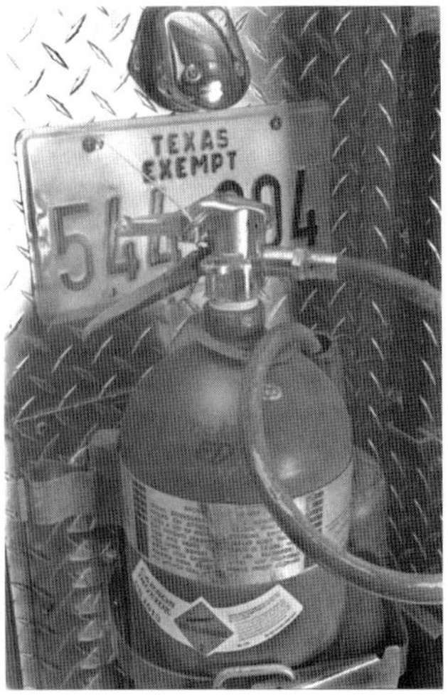
TEXAS
EXEMPT

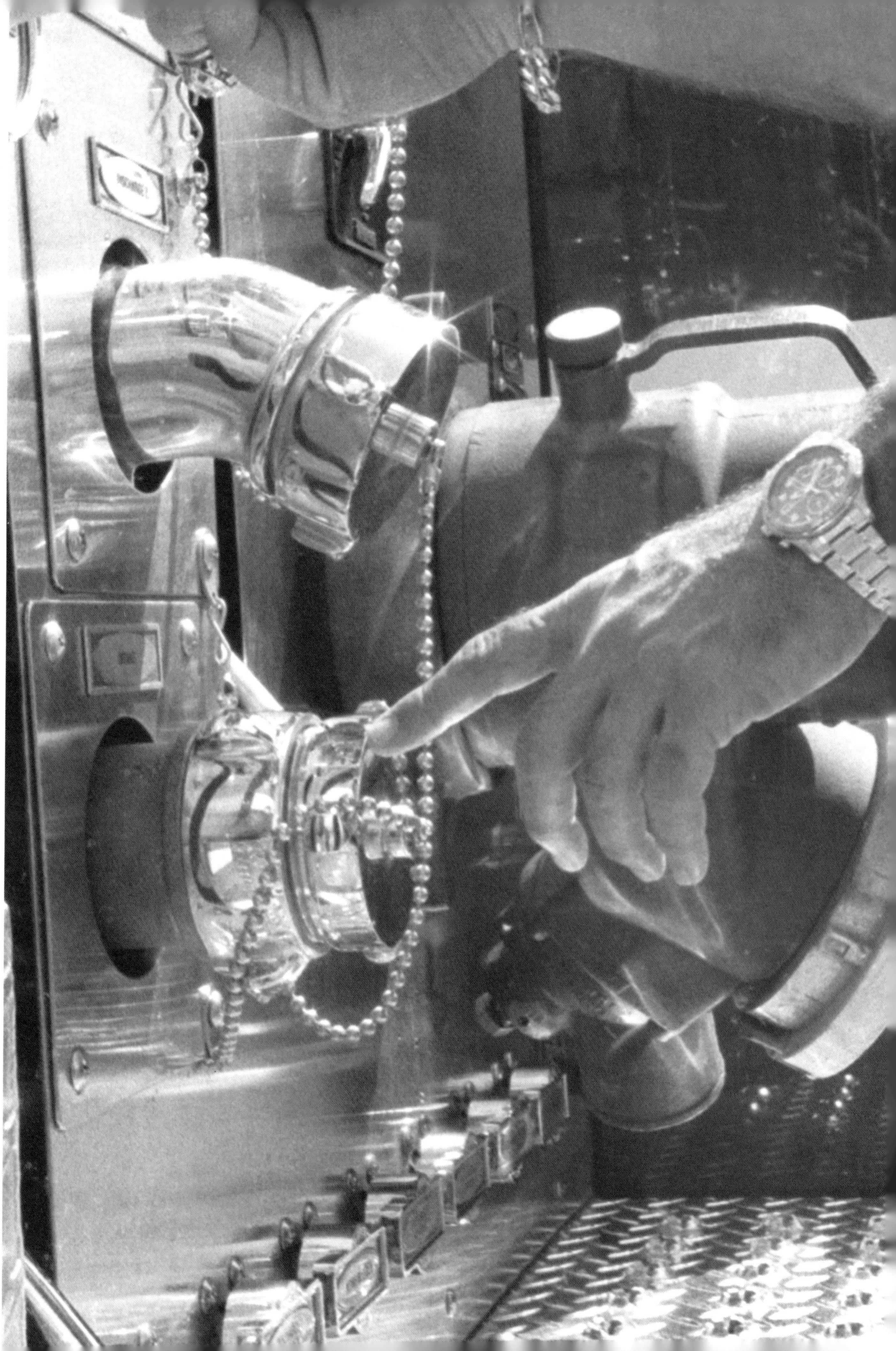

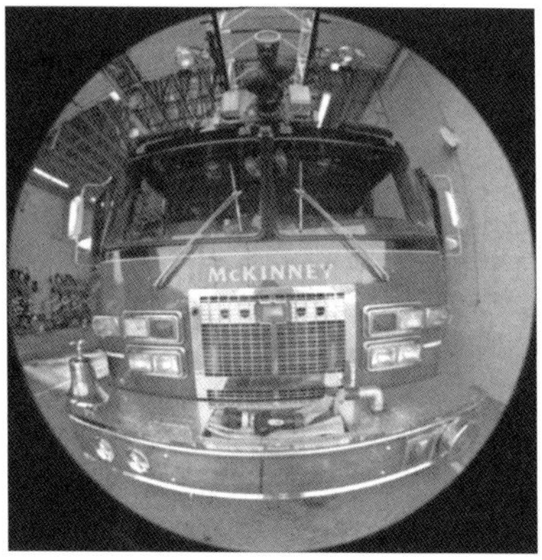
McKINNEY

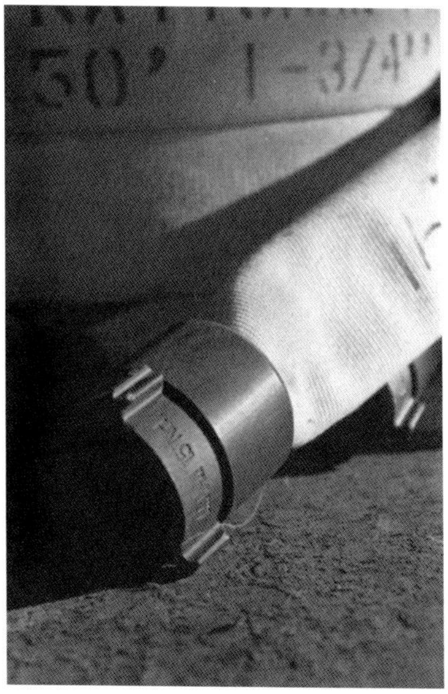
50' 1-3/4"

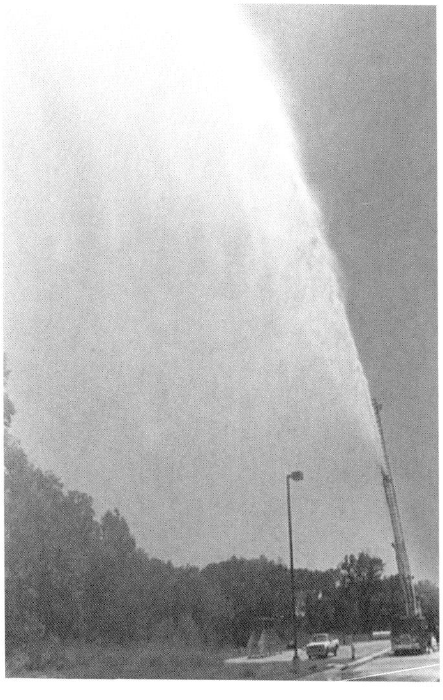

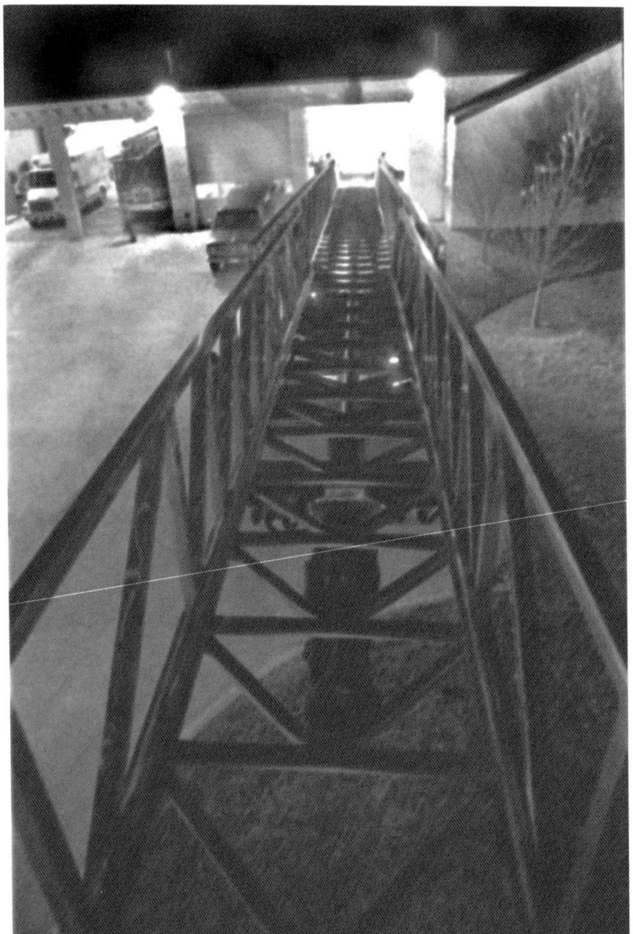

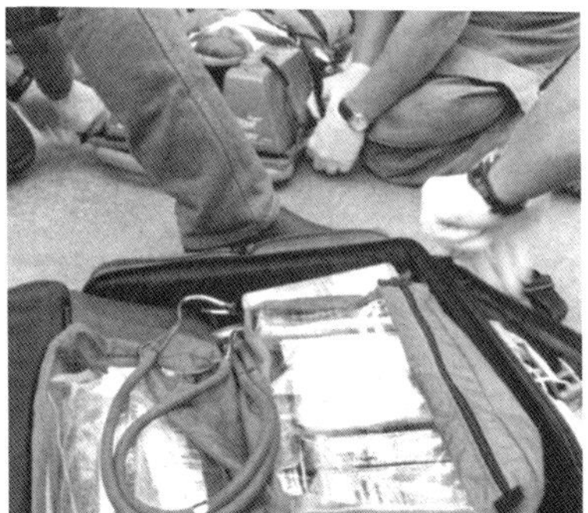

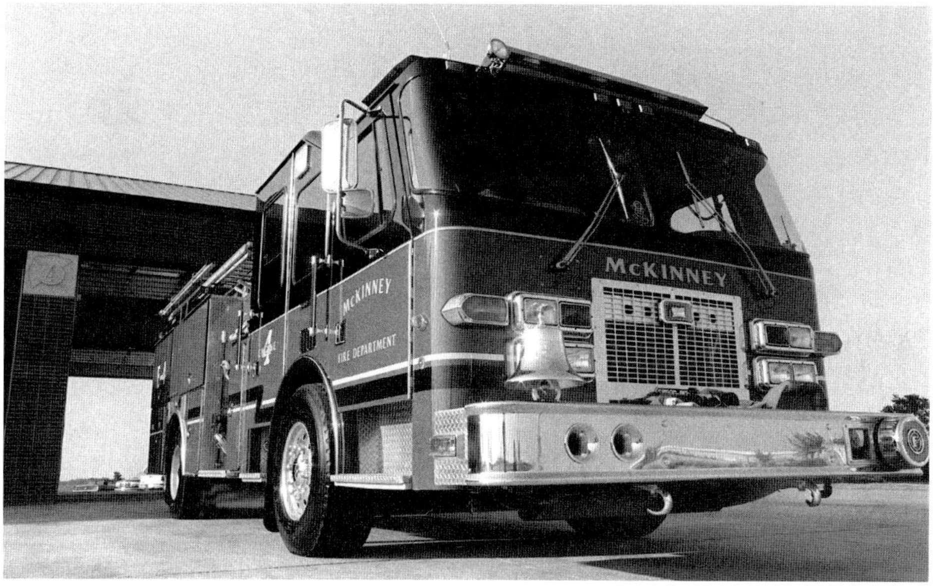
McKINNEY
McKINNEY
FIRE DEPARTMENT

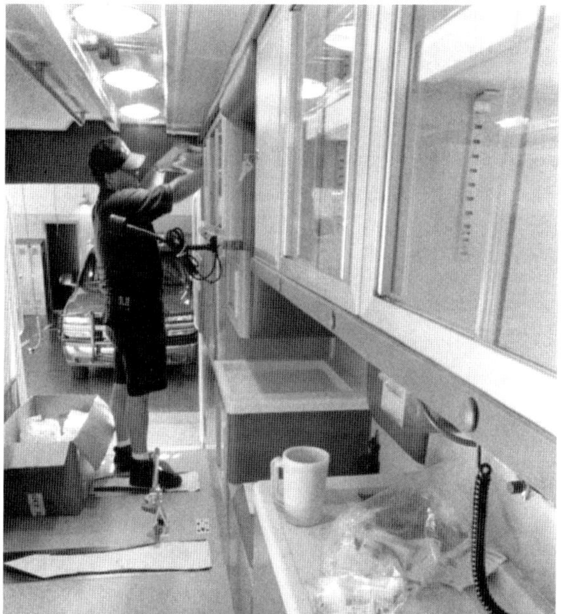

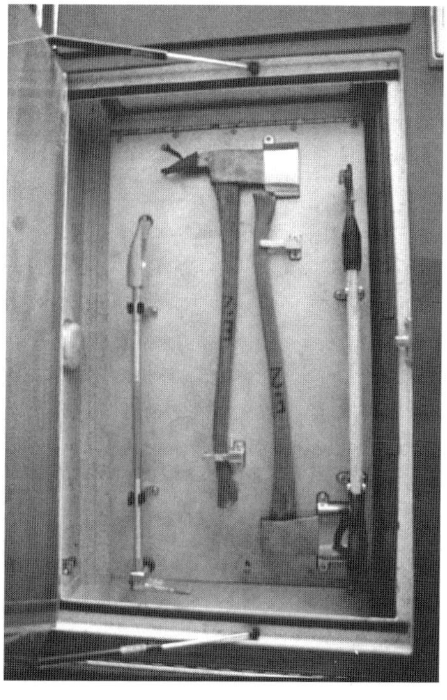

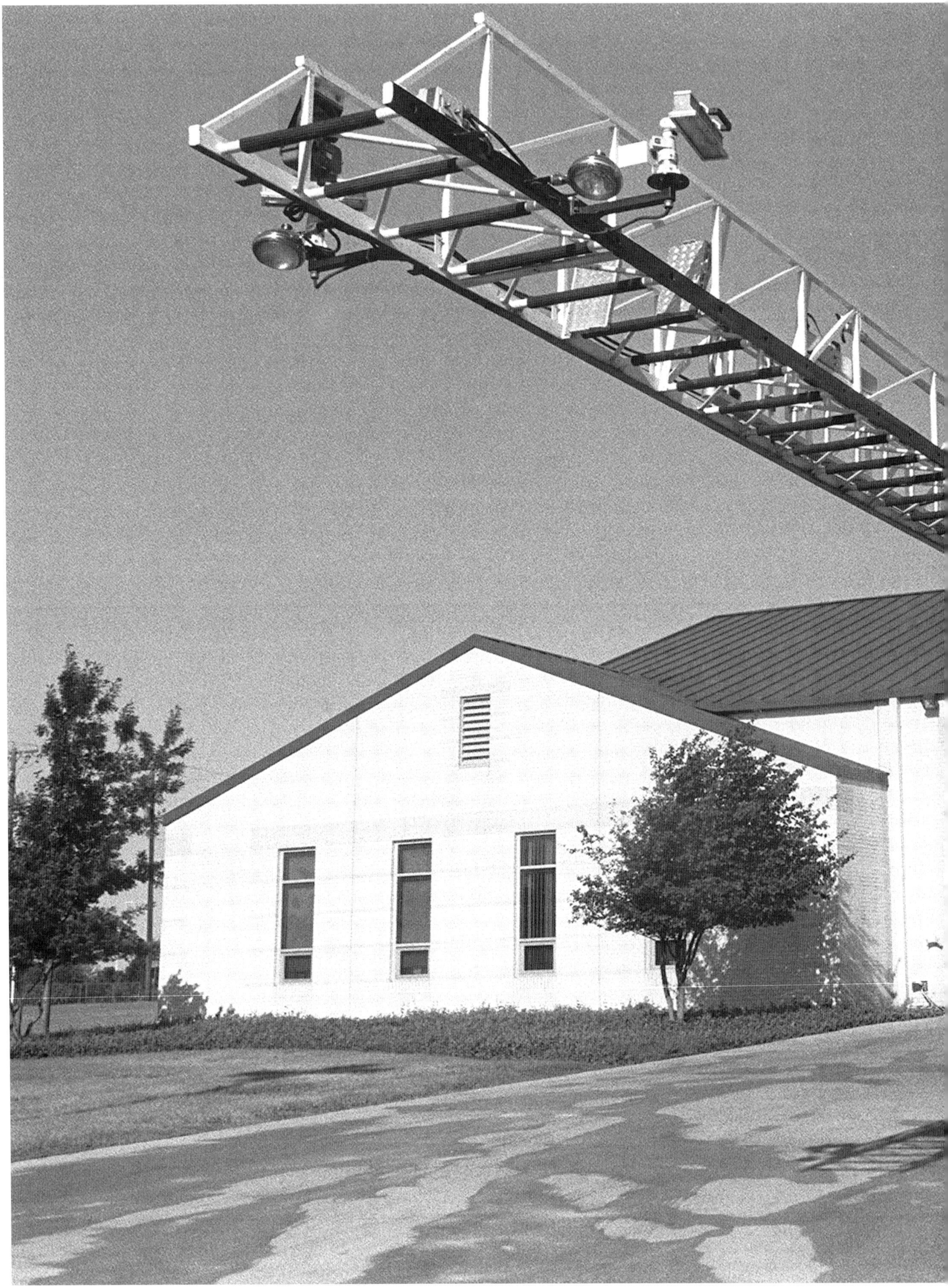

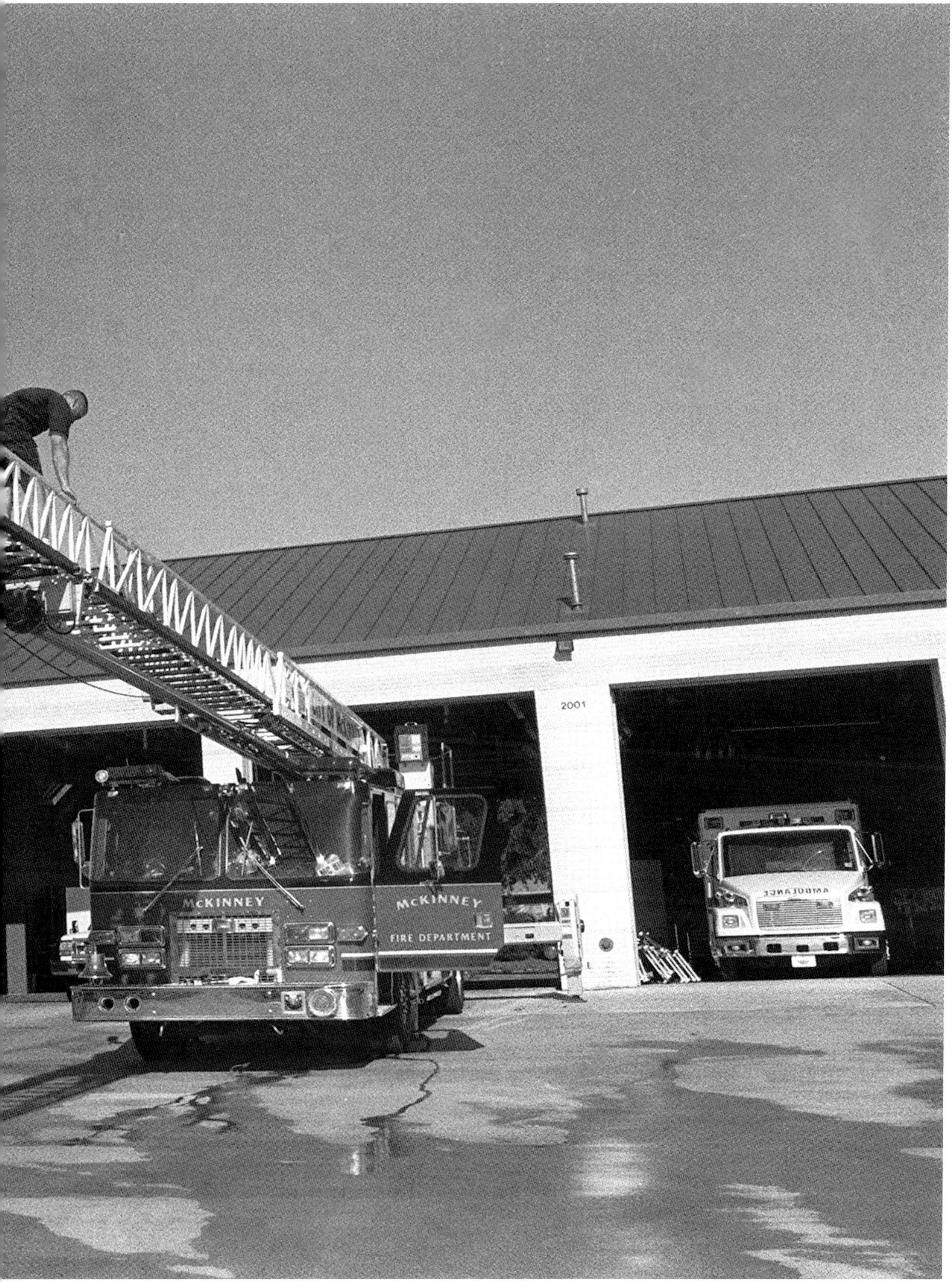
2001
McKINNEY
McKINNEY
FIRE DEPARTMENT

# community

What is a community without its fire department? Not only is it at the mercy of the beast, it is also without all the other benefits and civic contributions a fire department makes.

Remember the funny clowns who put on the fire prevention skit at your elementary school? They were the local Firefighters contributing their off-time to make fire prevention education a reality. Ever attend a neighborhood block party where the fire engine pulled up so that you and your friends could excitedly climb all over it? Guess who wished they were there with their family. Guess who polished the bright red monster back to shiny brilliance after all the sticky popsicle fingers went home? You've got it.

The list of community contributions goes on and on, but just as most Firefighters do not talk much about them, neither will I. It's part of their Silent Glory.

But, stop in some afternoon with your wife and kids at your local fire station, take a tour and say thanks to each of the Firefighters for all they do. It will be a thrill for everyone, especially the folks in the house. It's always really nice to hear you are truly appreciated... in person.

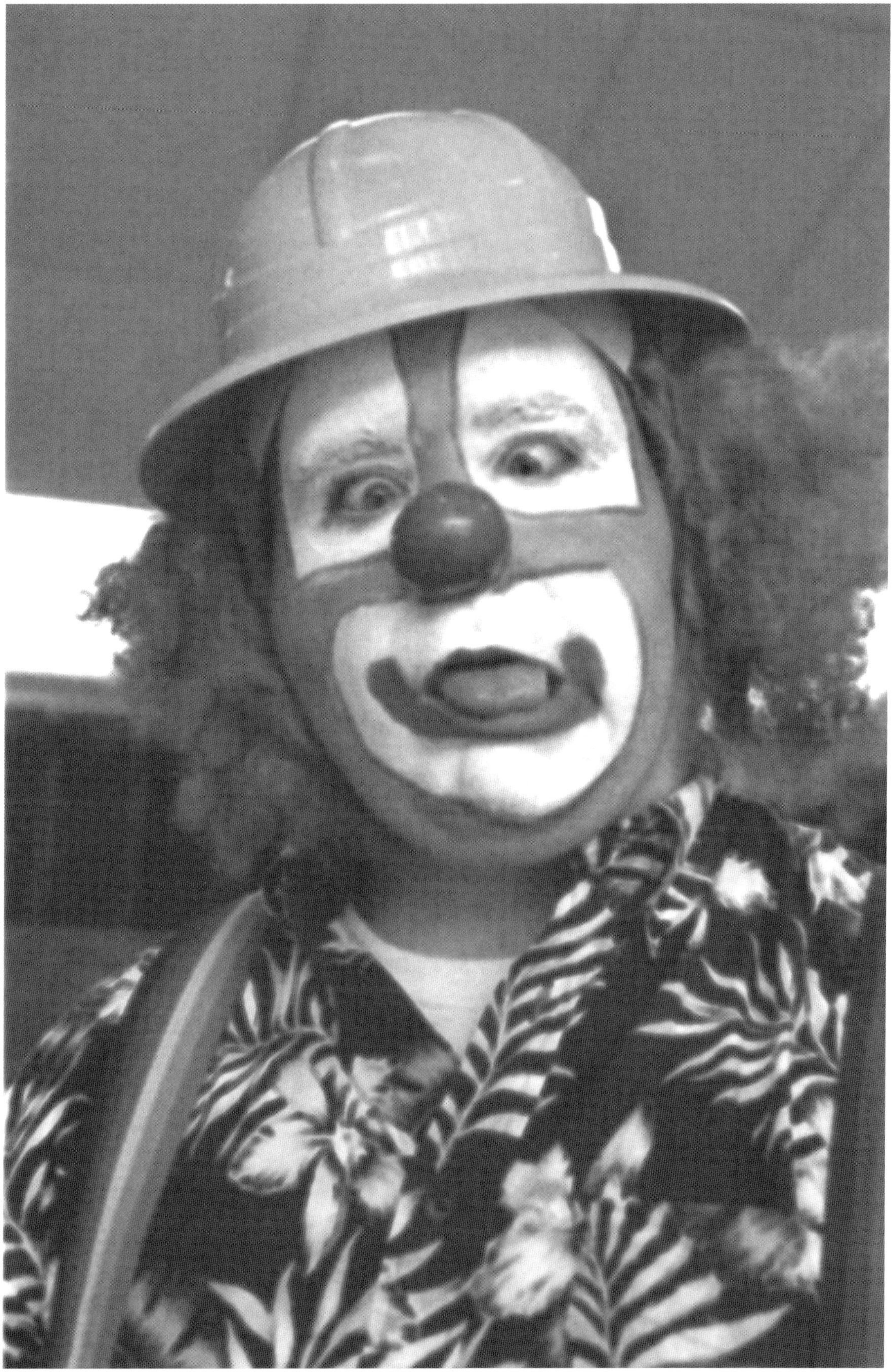

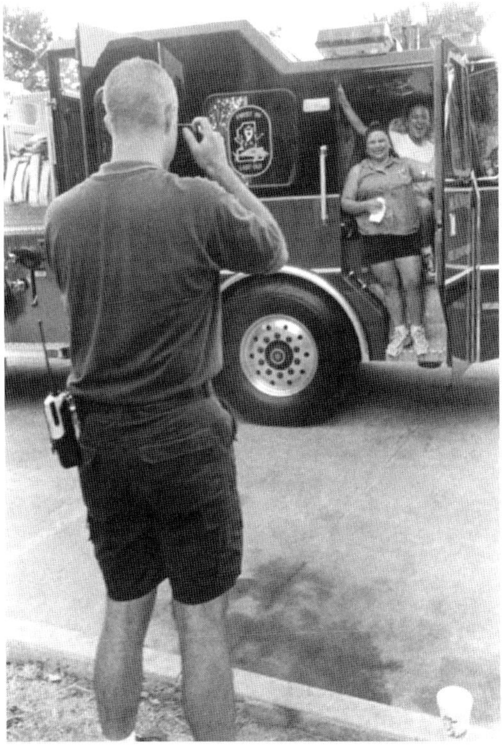

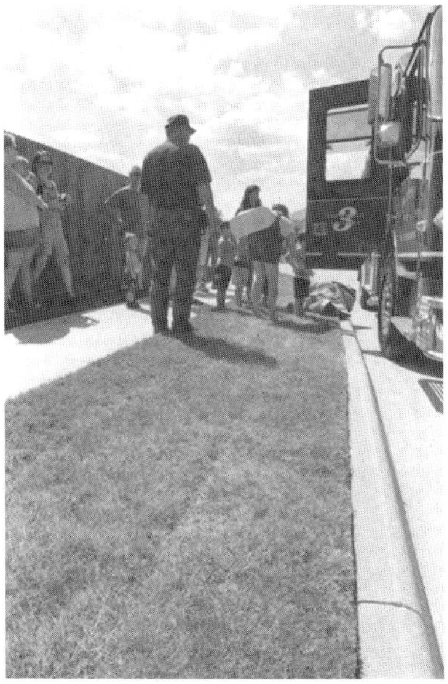

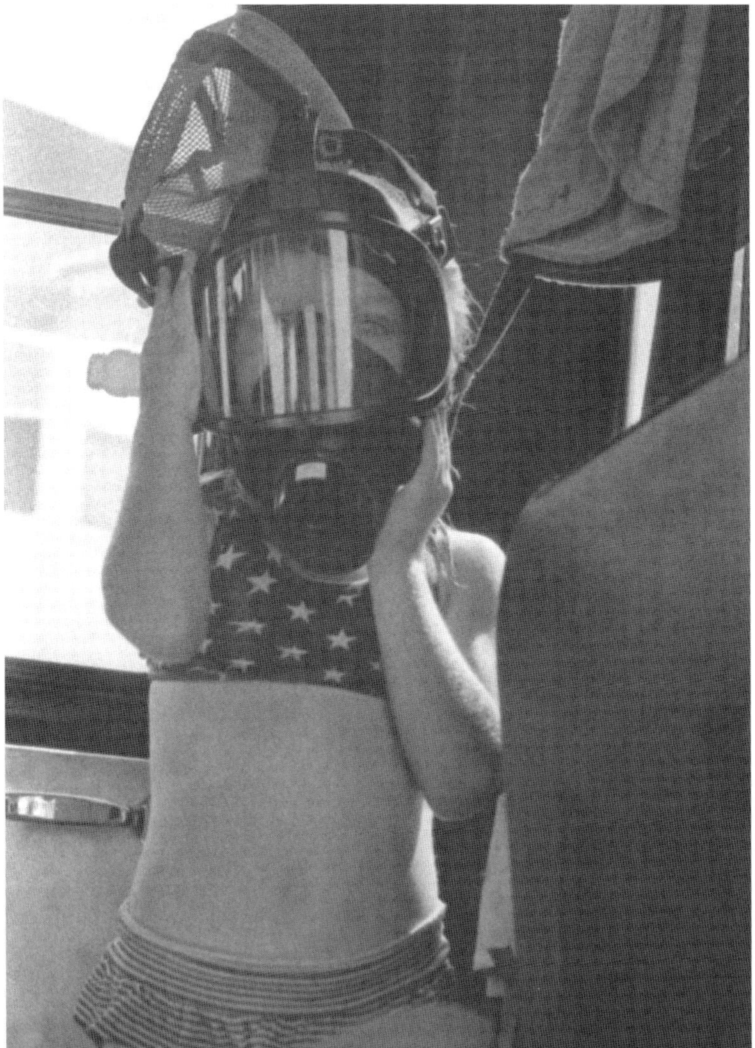

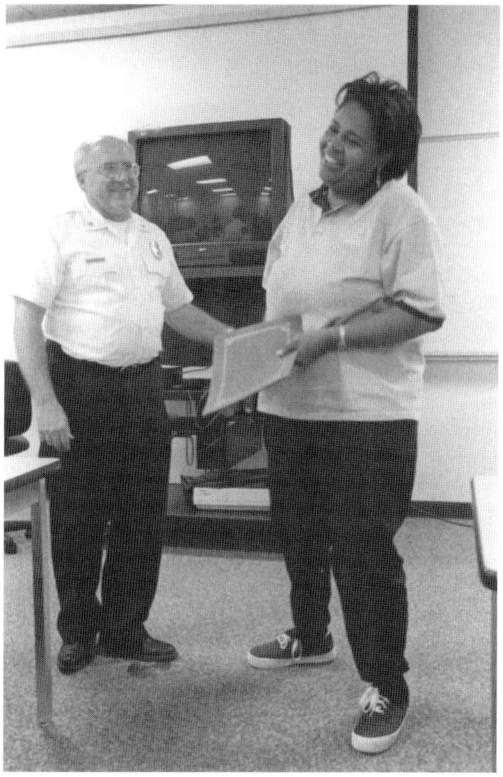

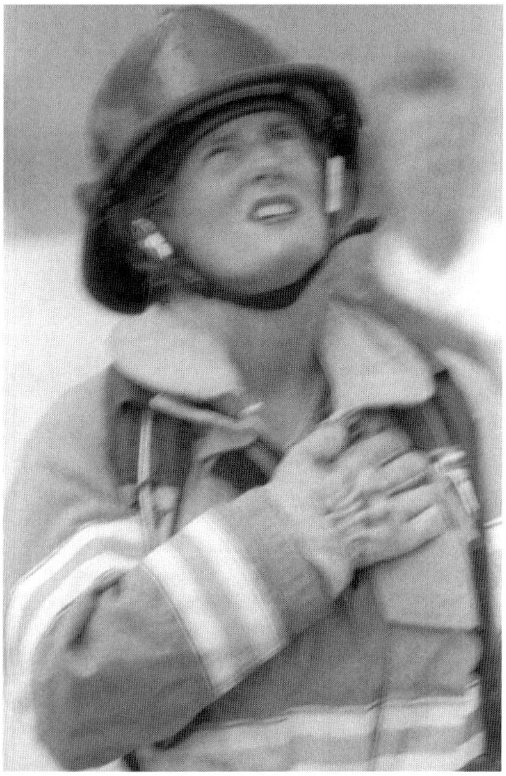

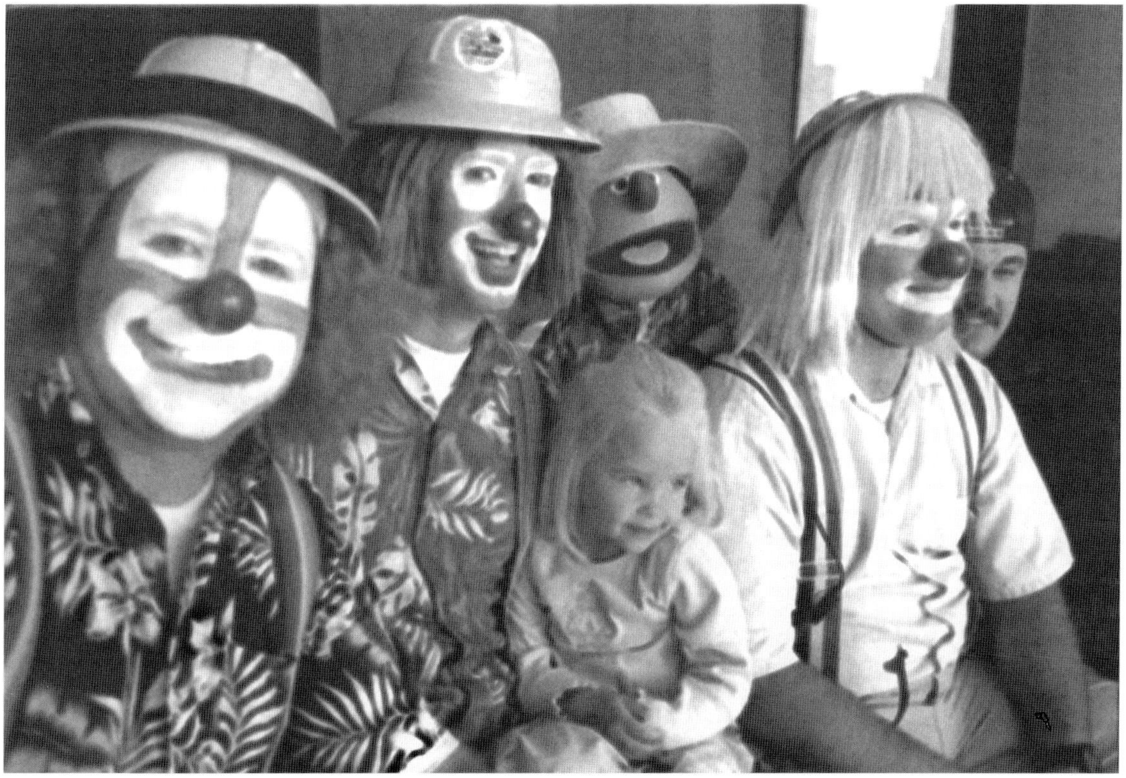

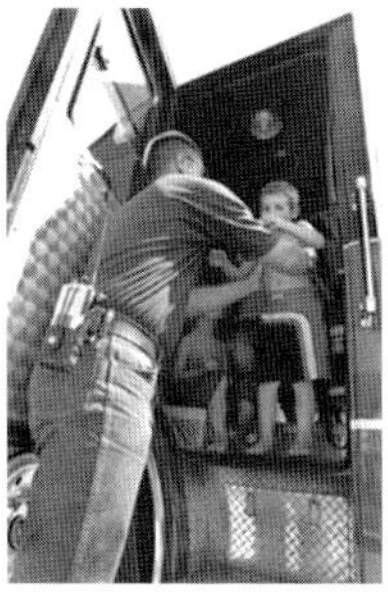

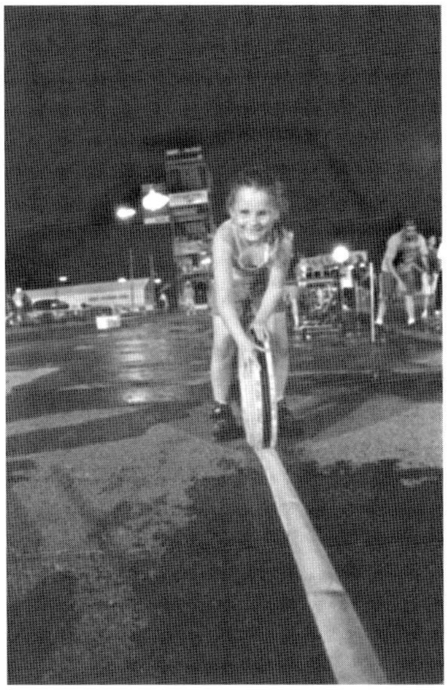

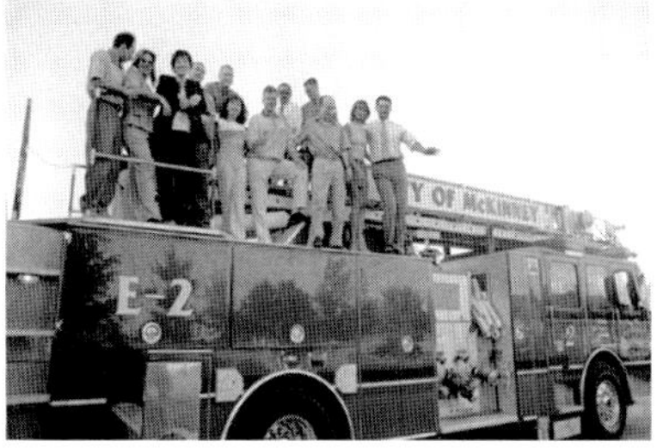
E-2

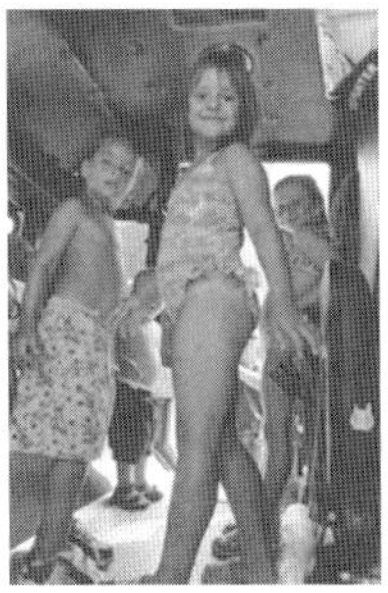

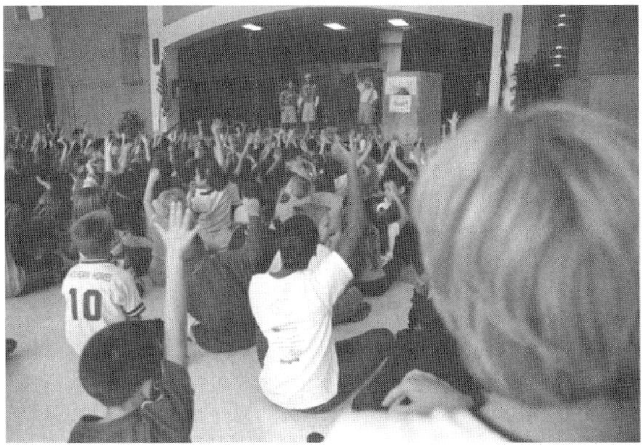

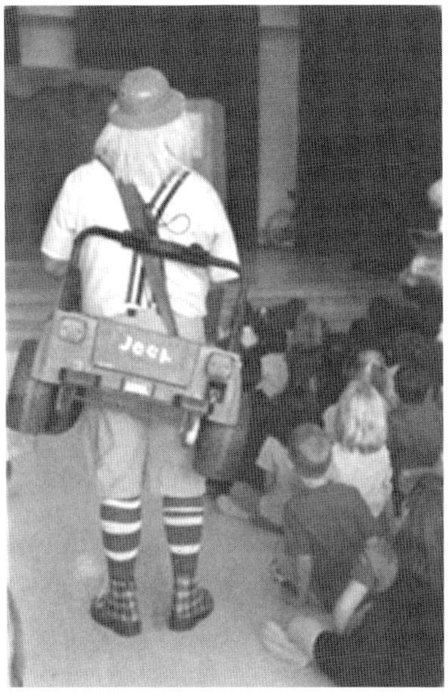
Jeep

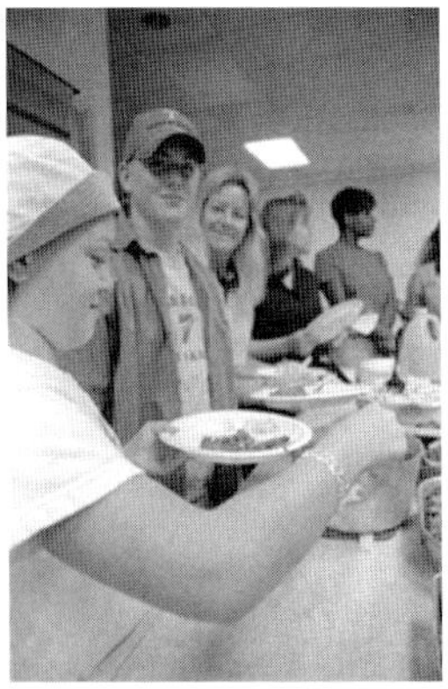

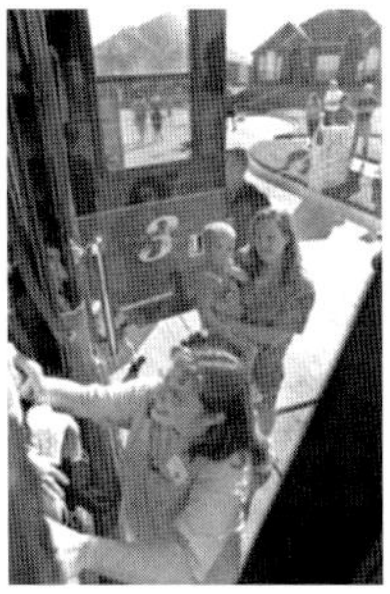

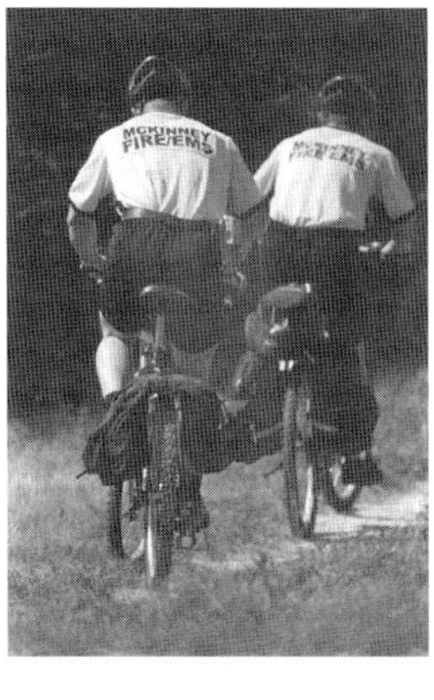
McKINNEY
FIRE/EMS

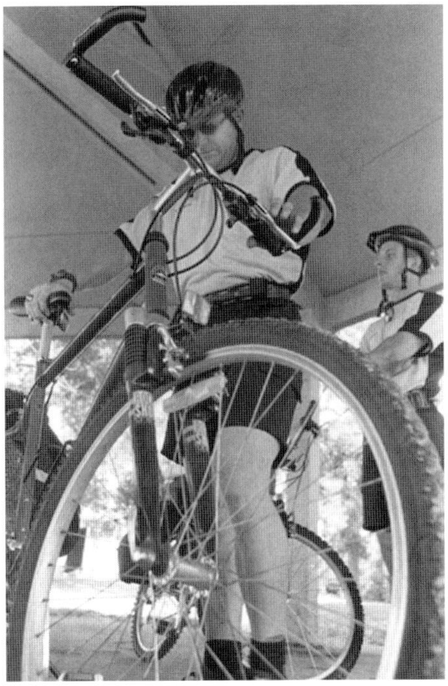

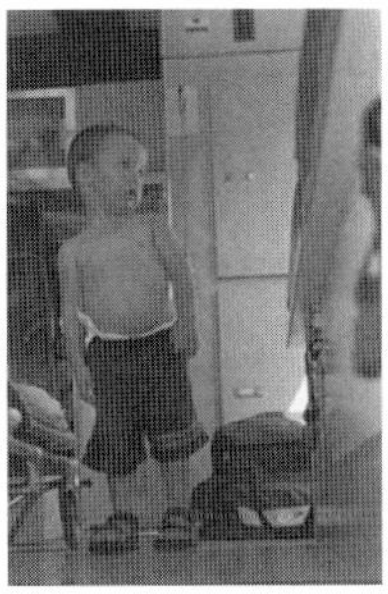

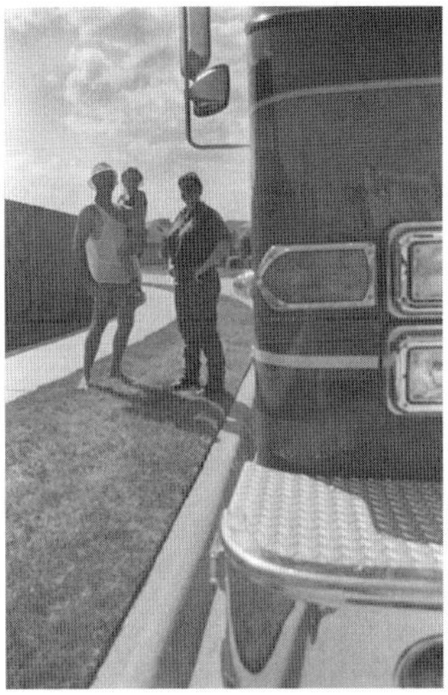

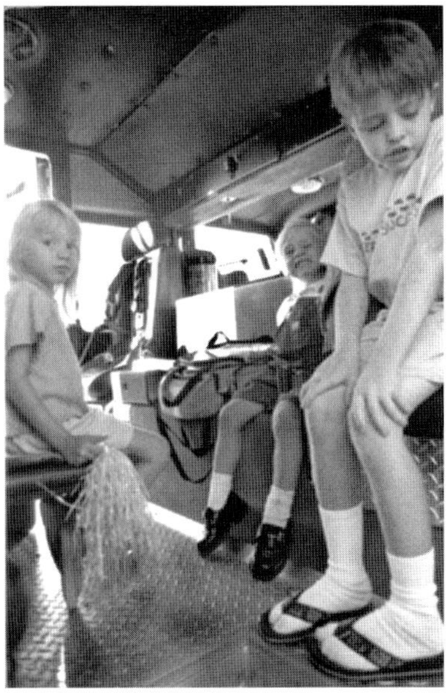

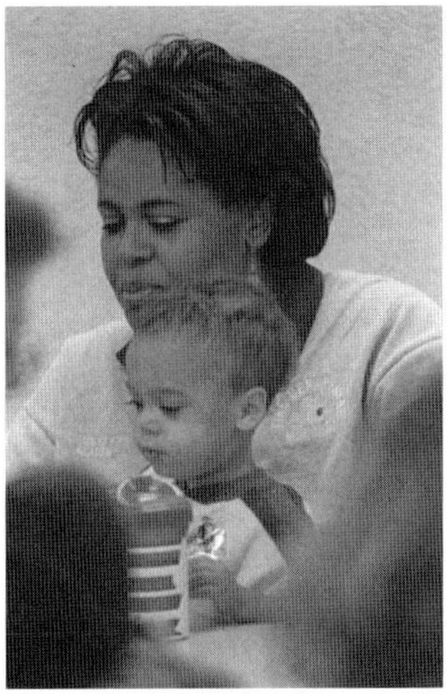

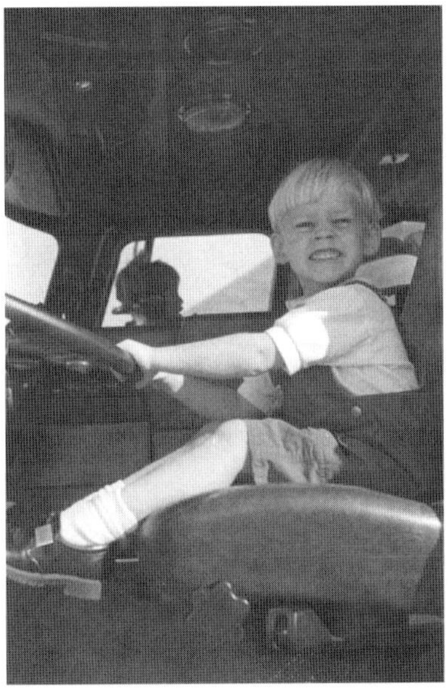

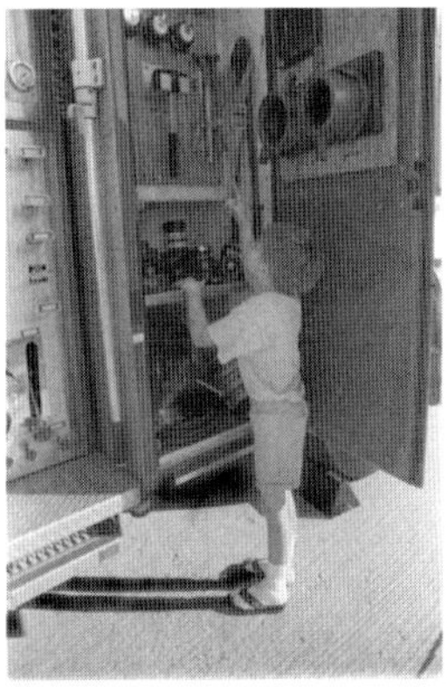

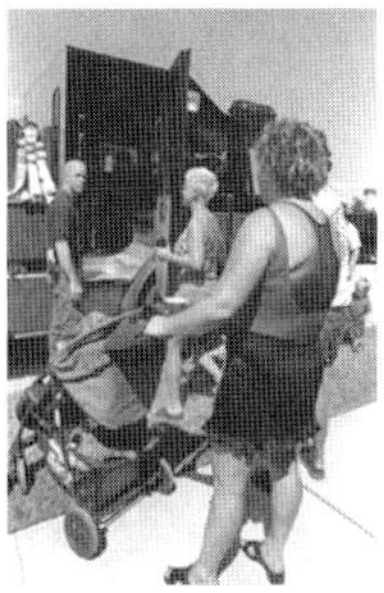

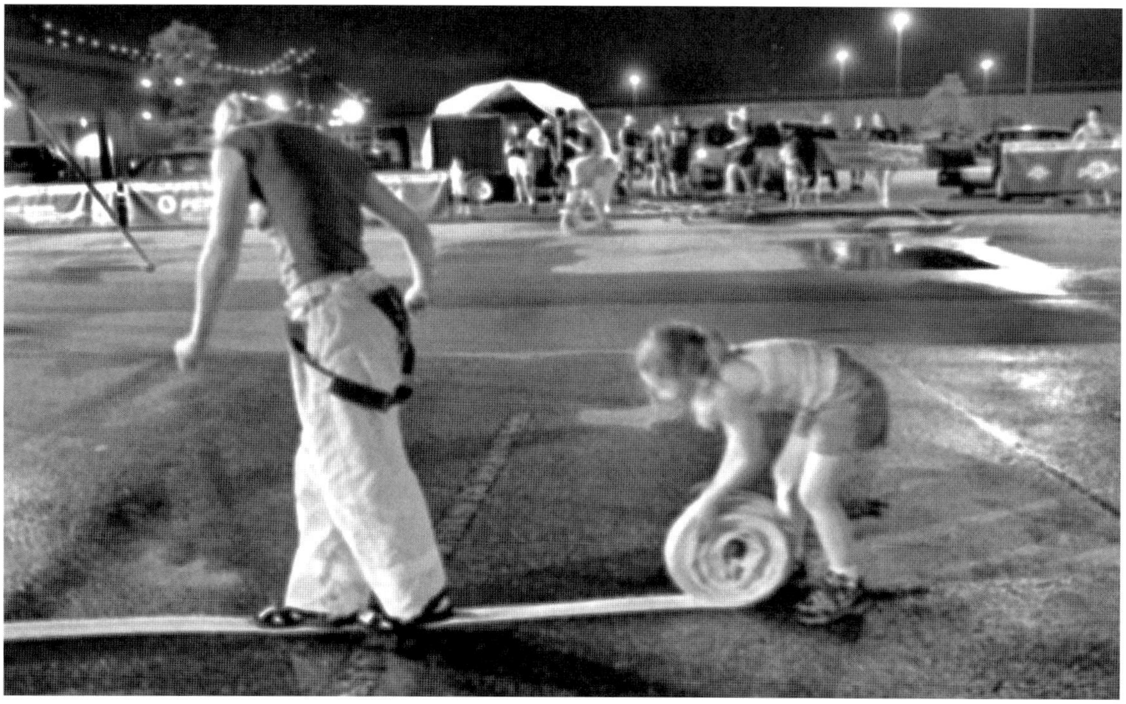

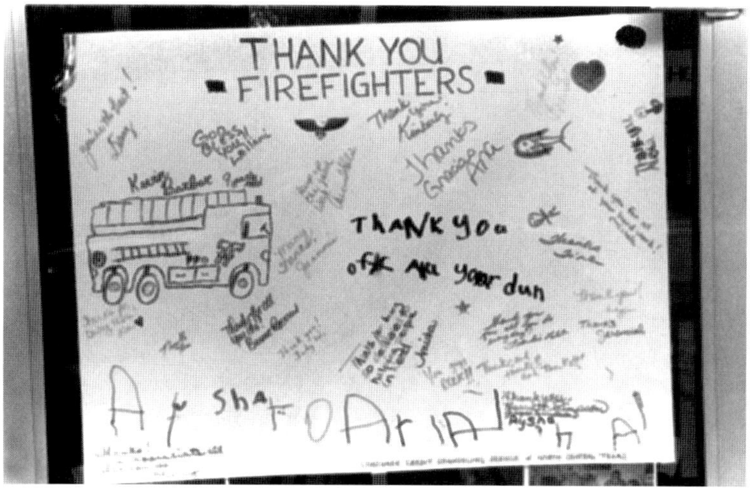
THANK YOU
FIREFIGHTERS
THANK you

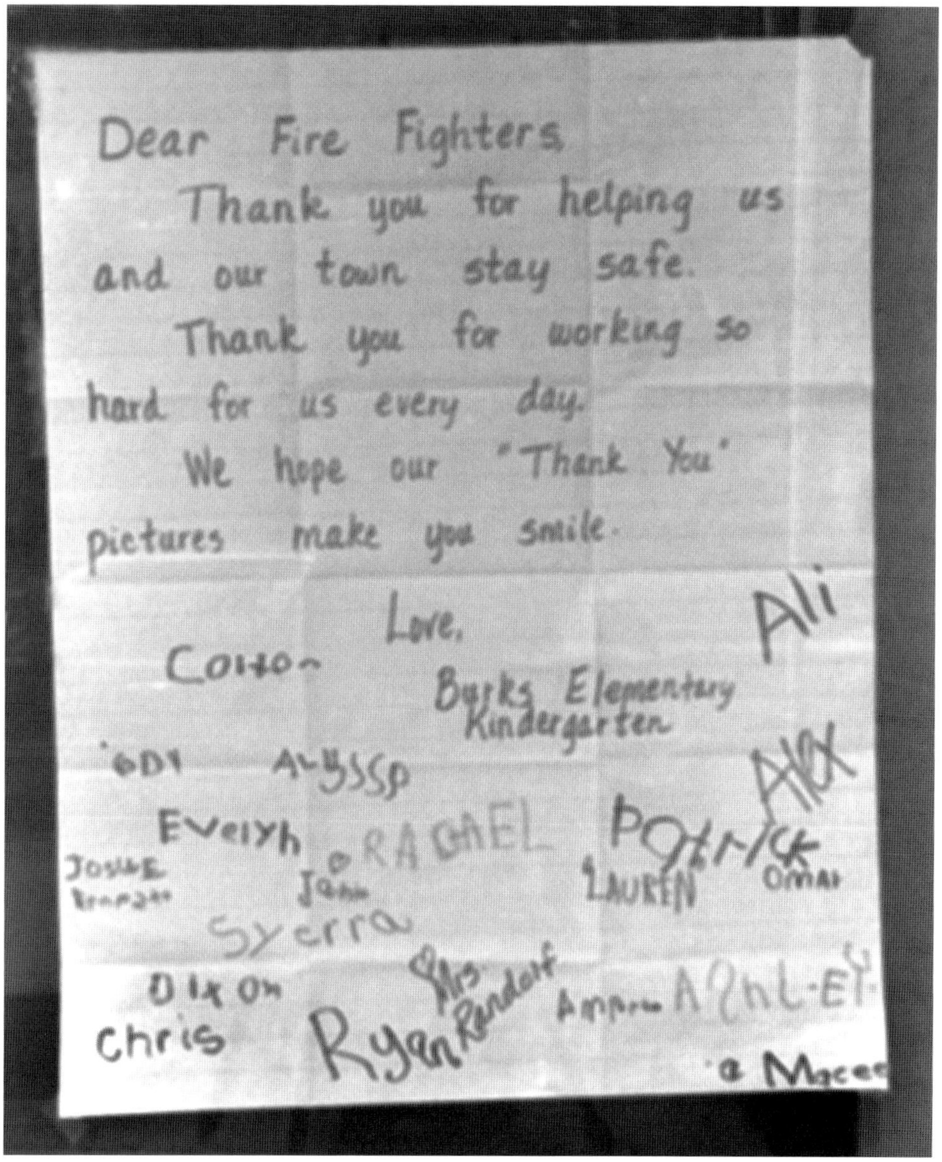
Dear Fire Fighters
Thank you for helping us
and our town stay safe.
Thank you for working so
hard for us every day.
We hope our "Thank You"
pictures make you smile.
Love,
Burks Elementary
Kindergarten
Ali
Alex
RACHEL
LAUREN
Syerra
Dixon
Chris
Ryan

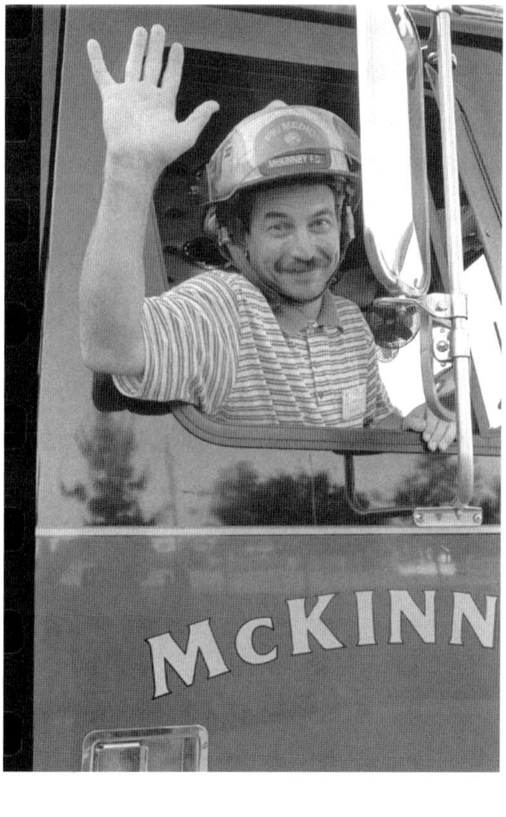
McKINN

# family

If you are a Firefighter, you are in a unique and special international family. Membership is an honor that is respected and held in highest regard by those priveleged to be a brother or sister. It is a real love and recognition for each other that is part of every member of the world wide corps of Firefighters regardless of country, color, faith, gender, language, age, positon, rank, or any characteristic that would differentiate any Firefighter within the family.

Each member knows the perils, each shares the thrill of conquest, and each personally burdens the devastation of defeat... from the inside, as participant, not witness. The difference of doing battle in the arena vs spectating from the stands. They share the unwritten, unspoken, common bond of the brotherhood.

Enjoy this chapter as you visit the images... You will probably not recognize or personally know any of the men or women in the photographs, yet their faces will have a certain familiarity. Each represents and symbolizes one of their brothers and sisters who are the Firefighters in your home town.

I am sincerely honored to have had the opportunity to share in their kinship.

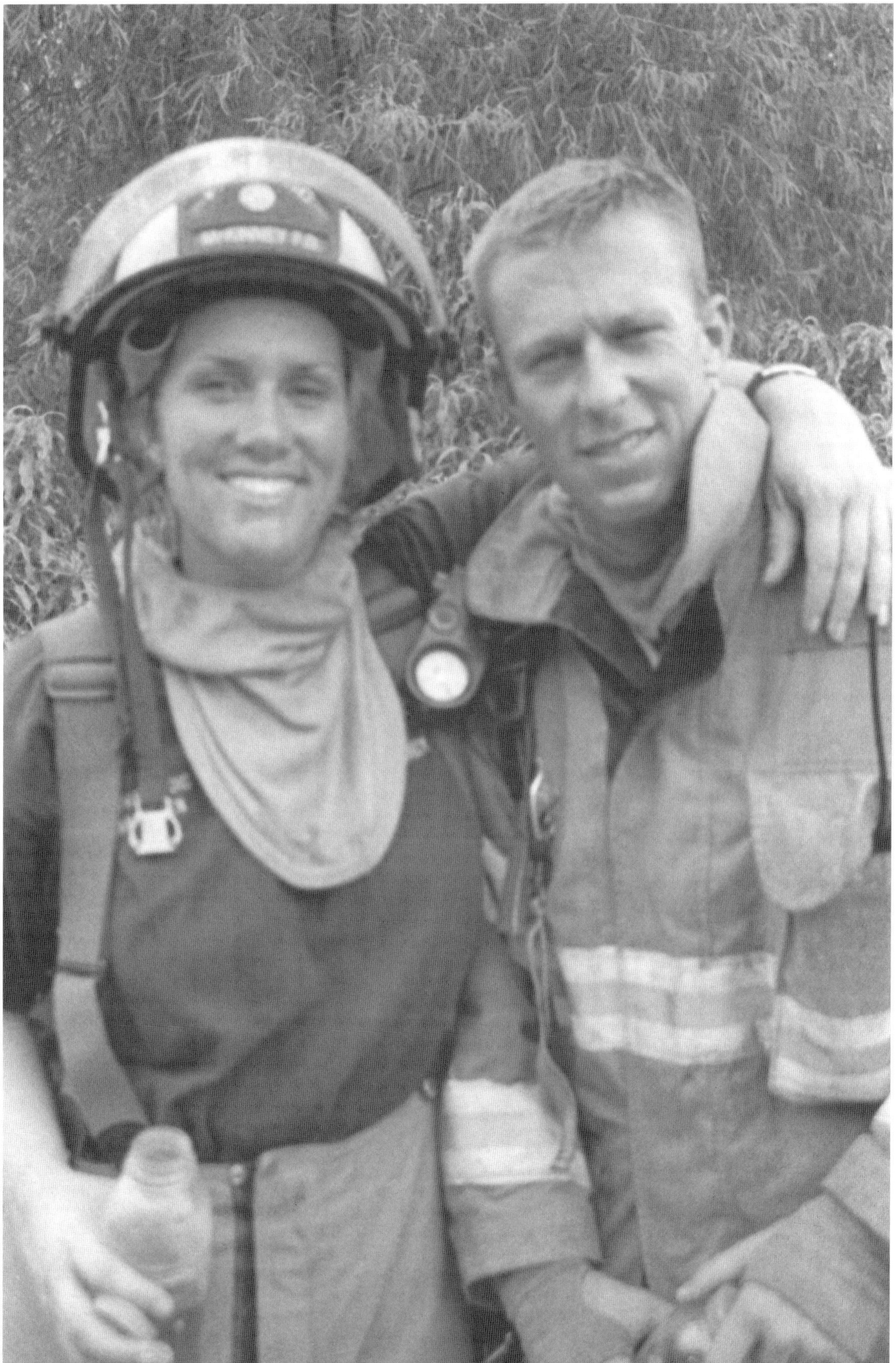

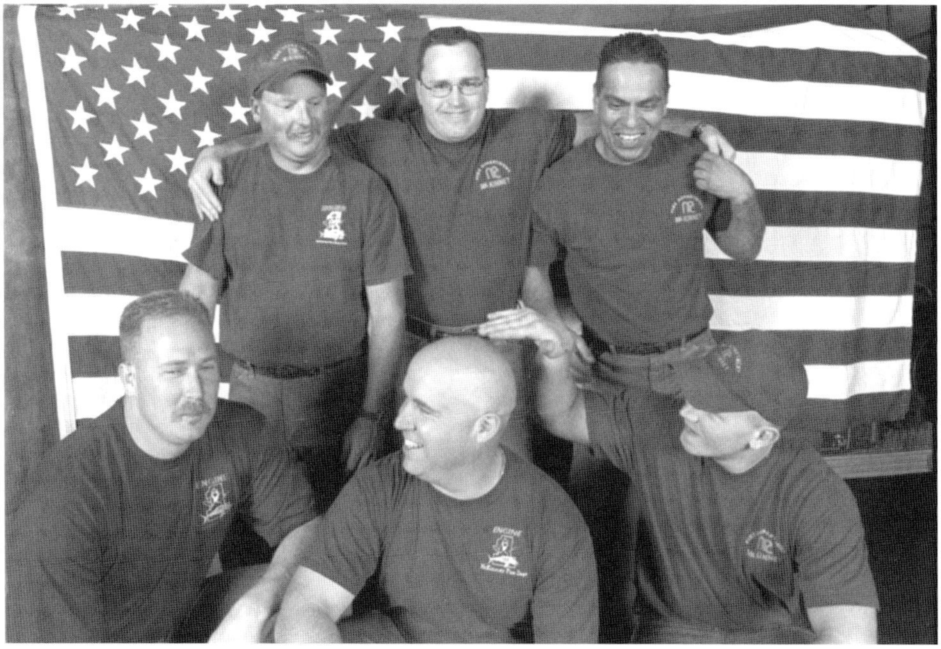

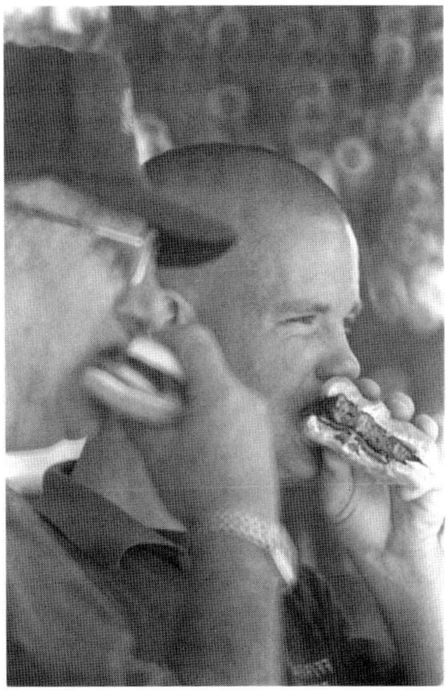

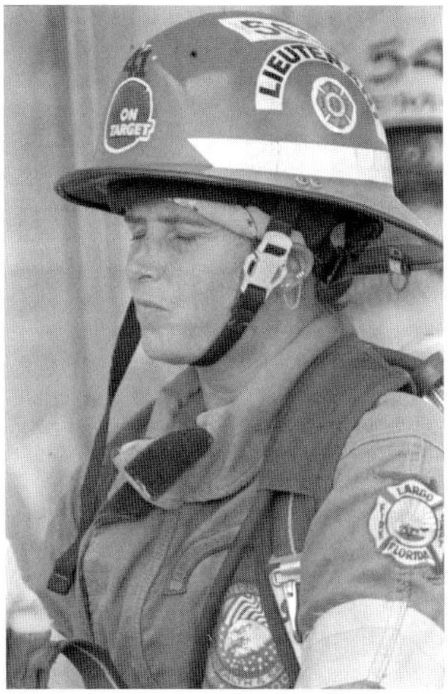
ON TARGET
LARGO
FLORIDA

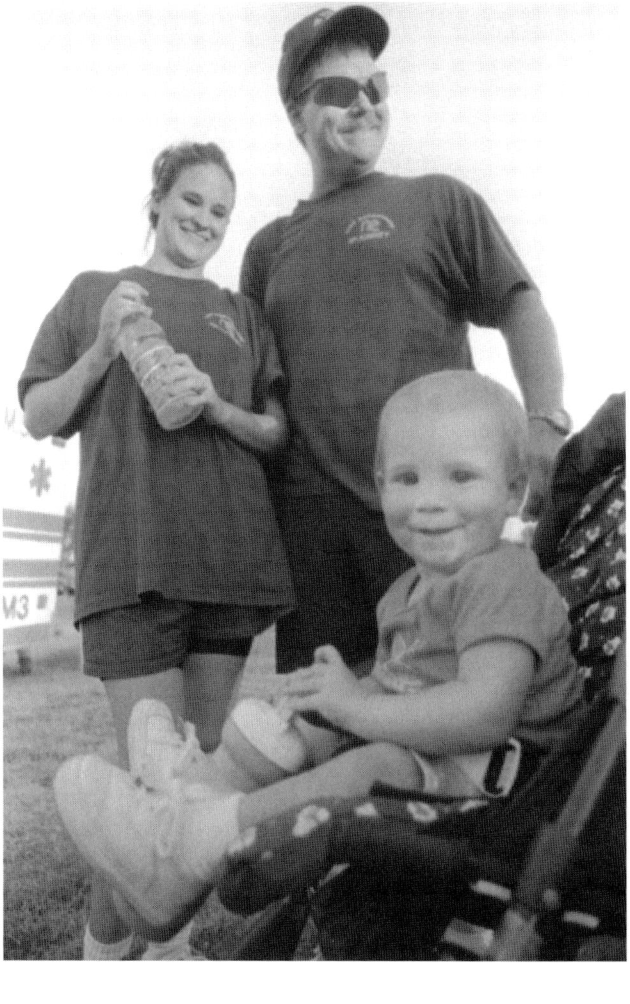

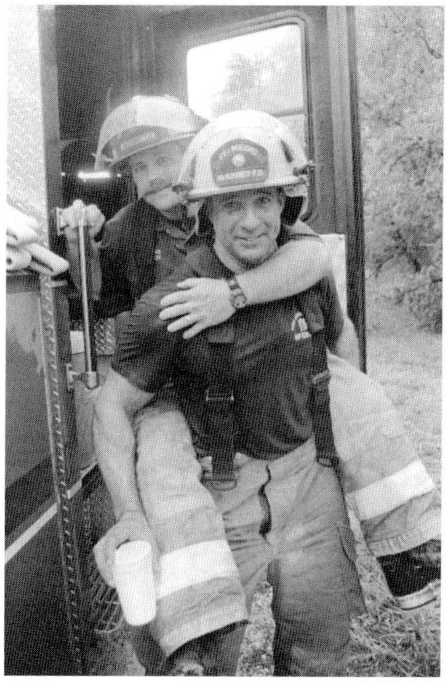

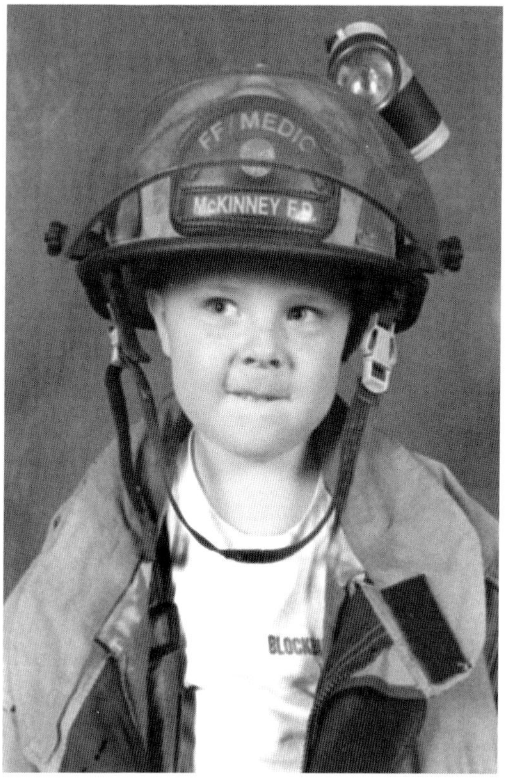
FF / MEDIC
McKINNEY F.D

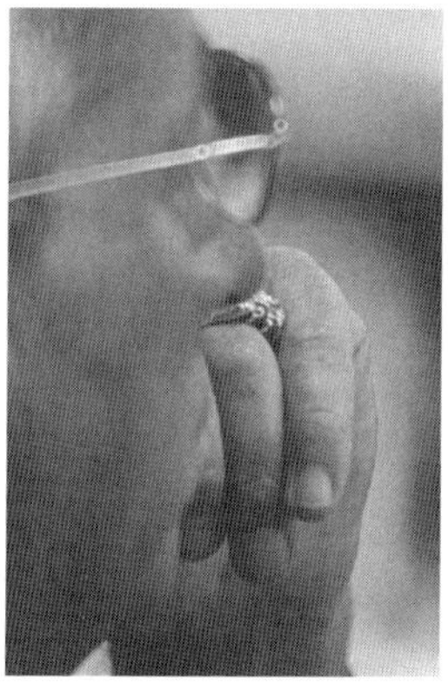

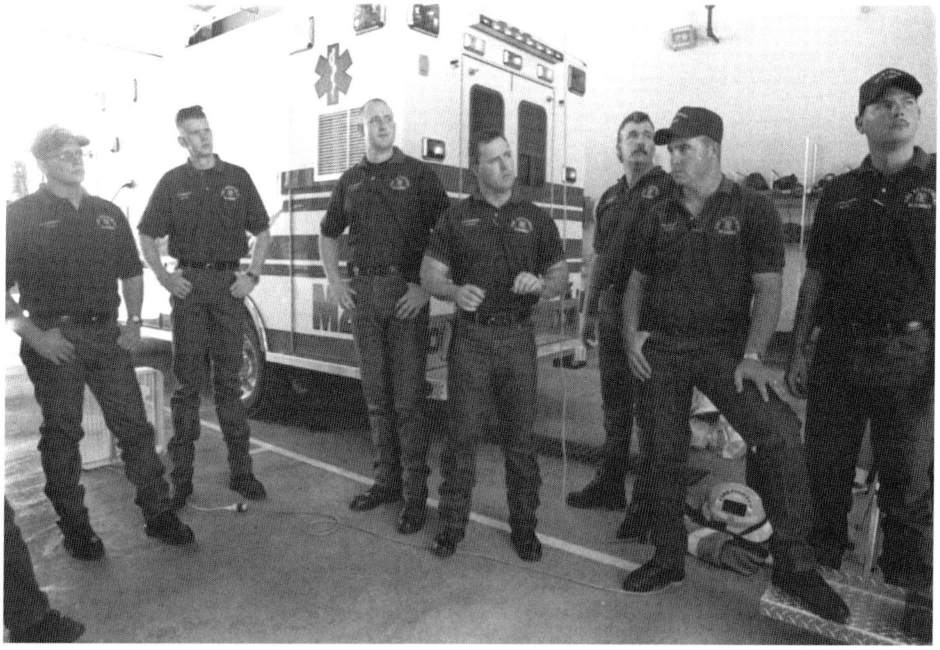

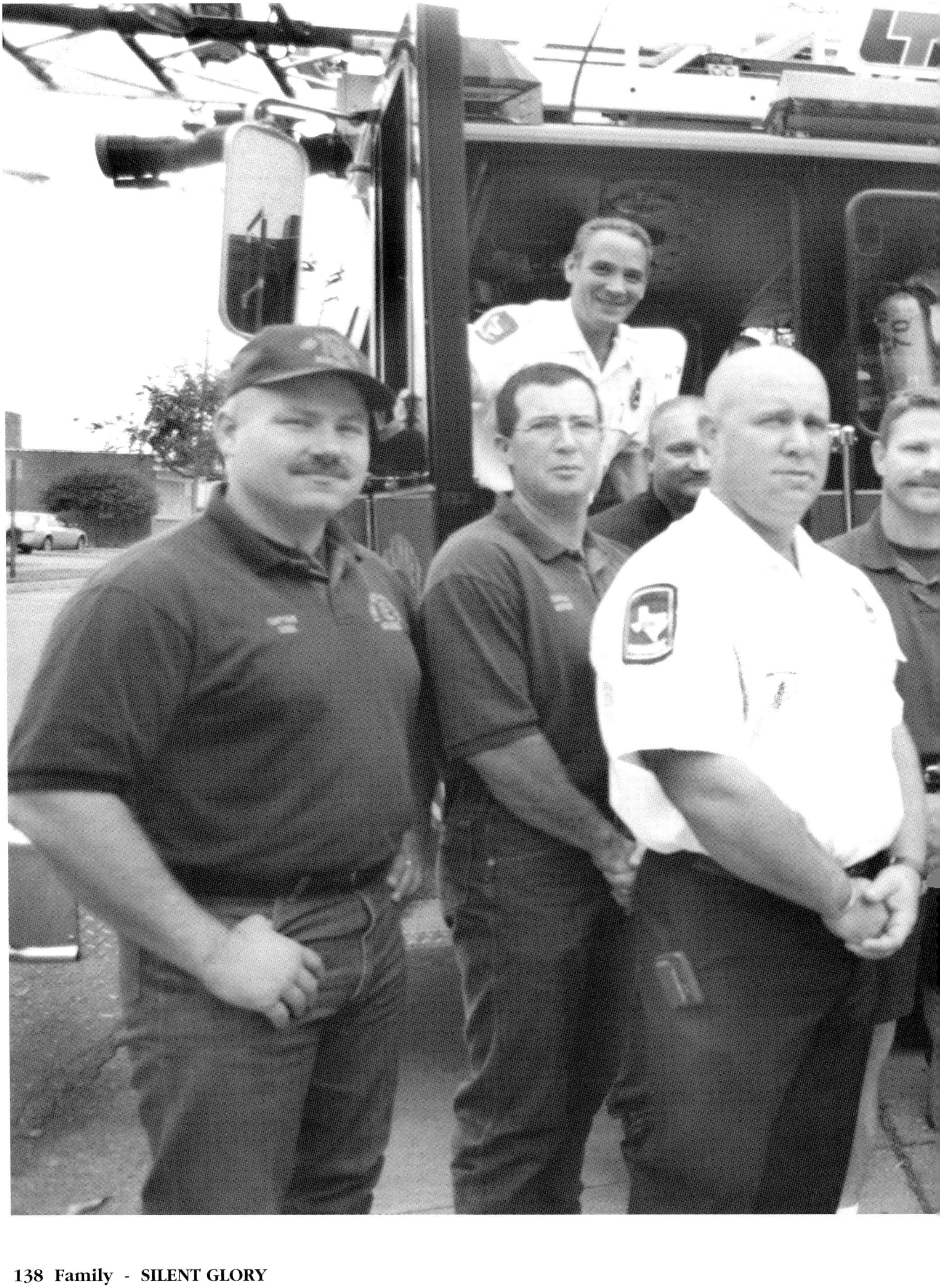

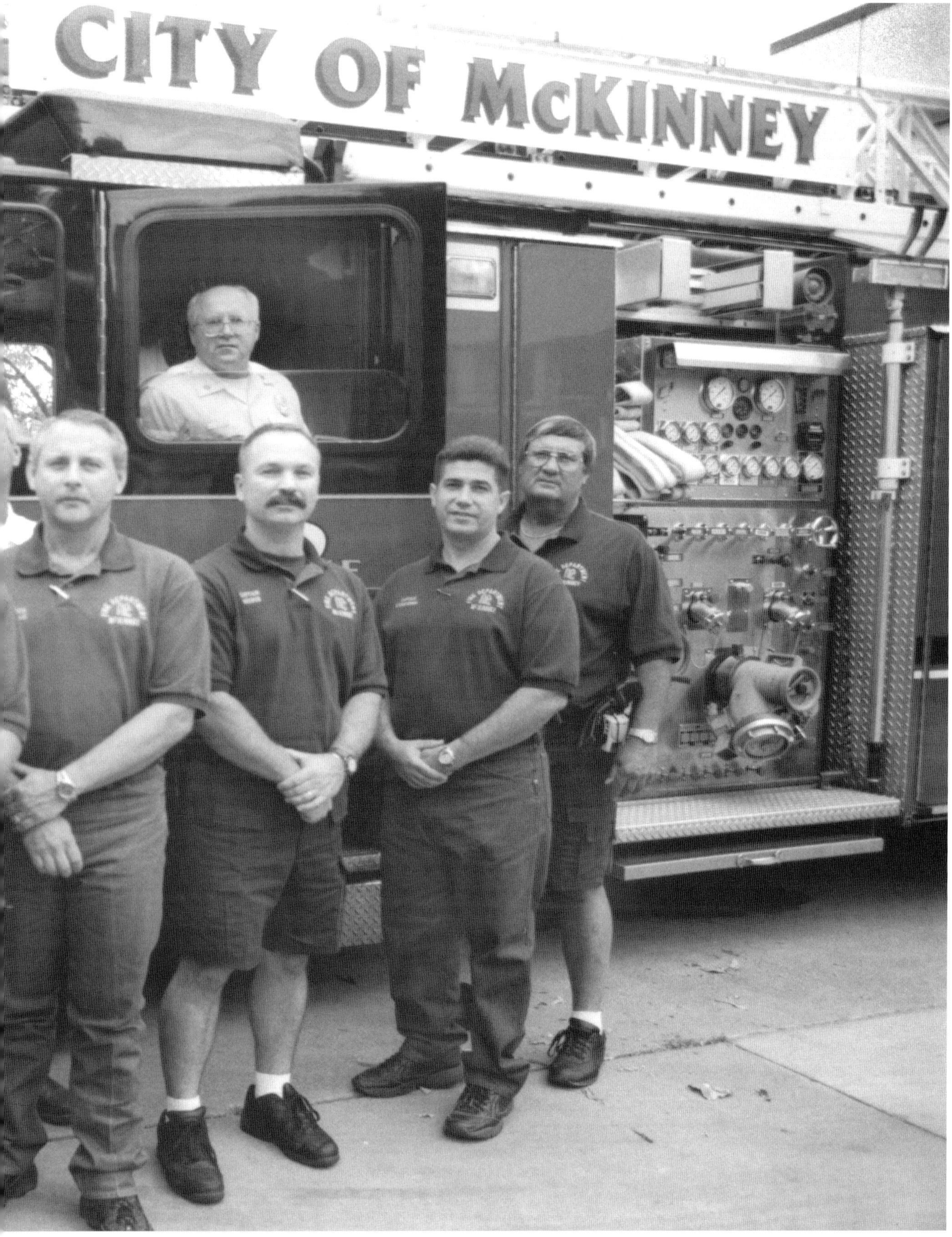
CITY OF McKINNEY

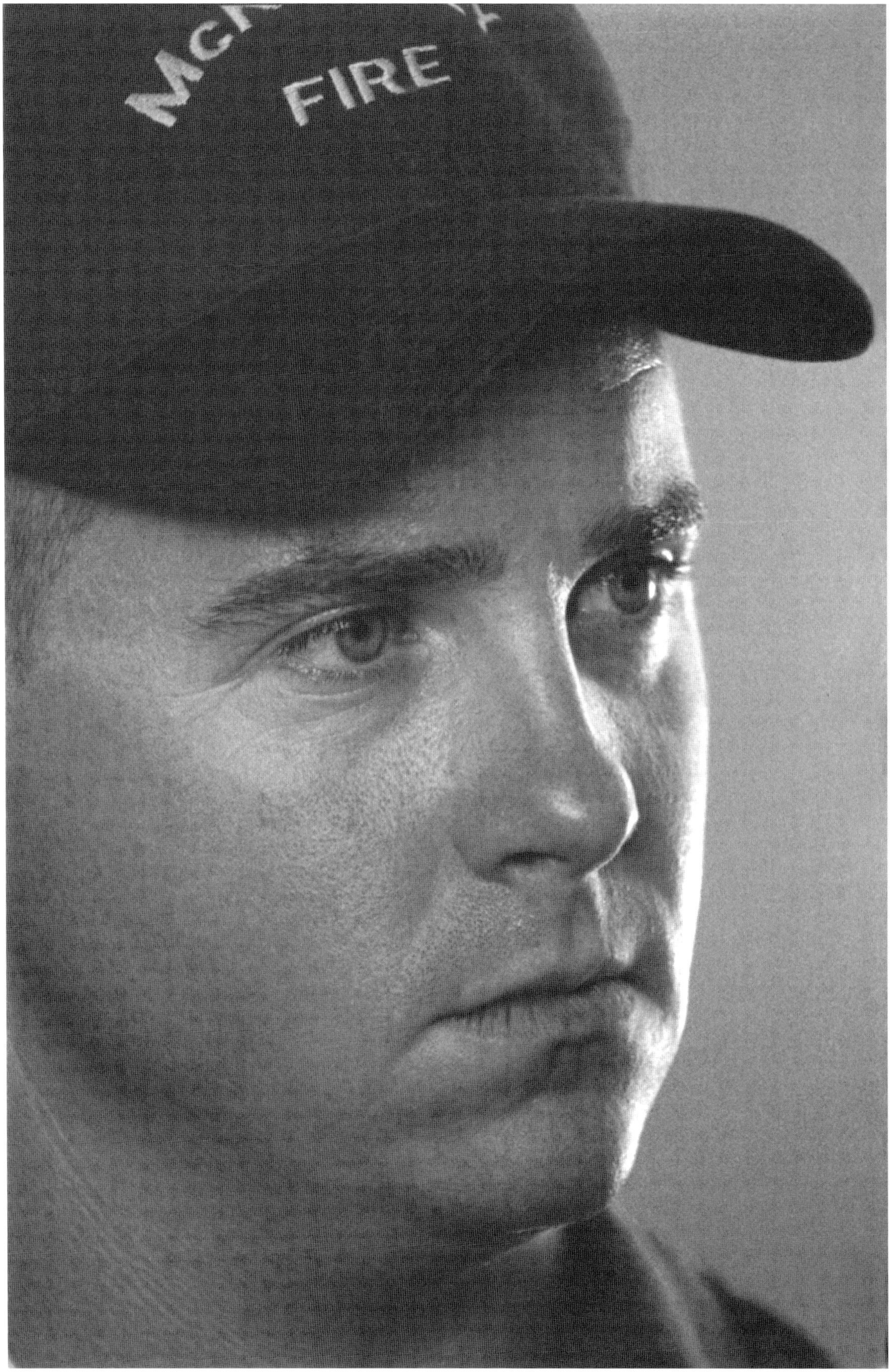
FIRE

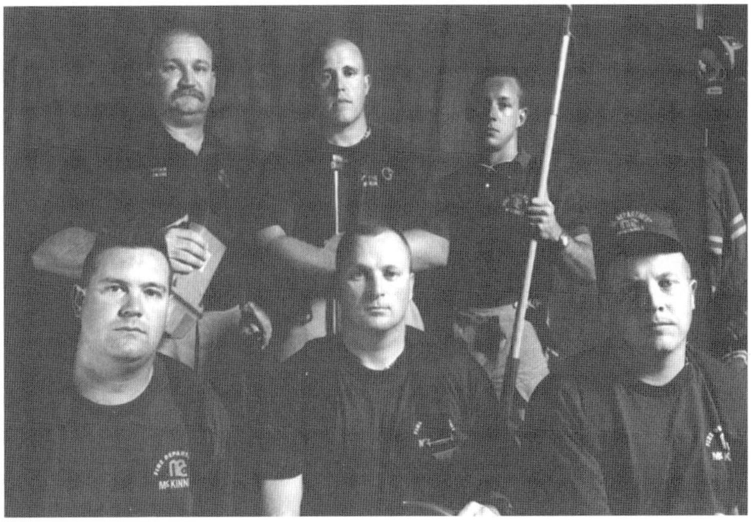

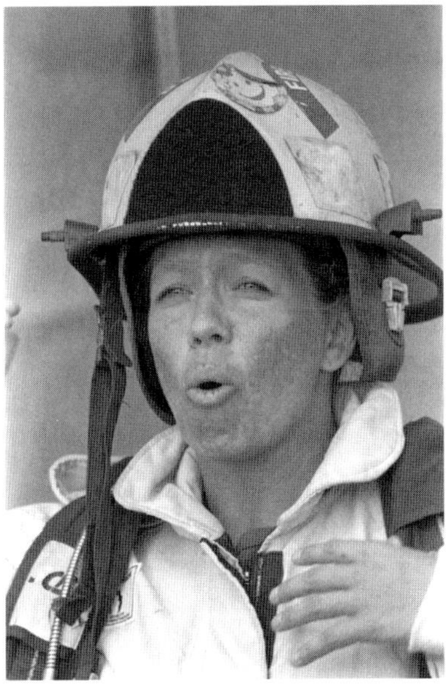

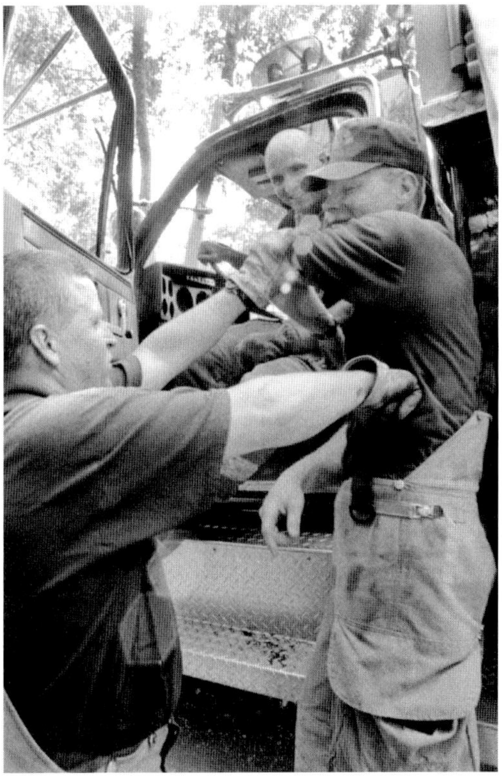

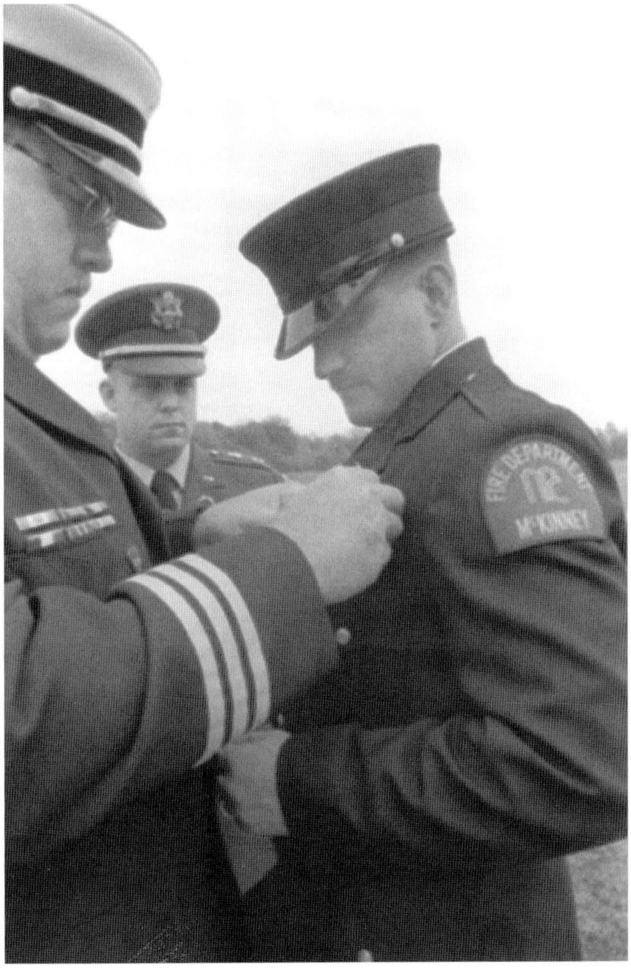
FIRE DEPARTMENT
McKINNEY

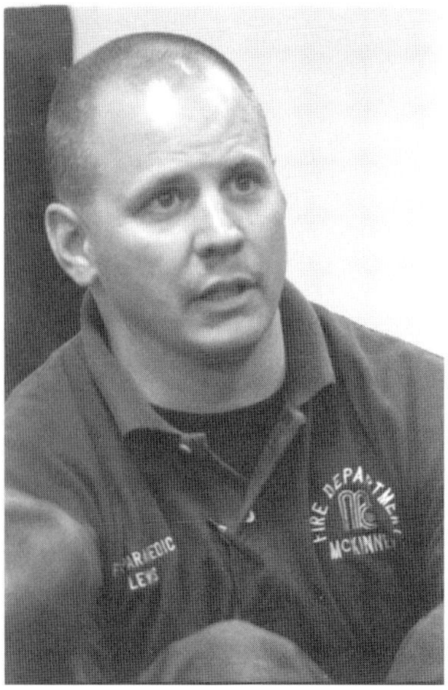
FIRE DEPARTMENT
McKINNEY

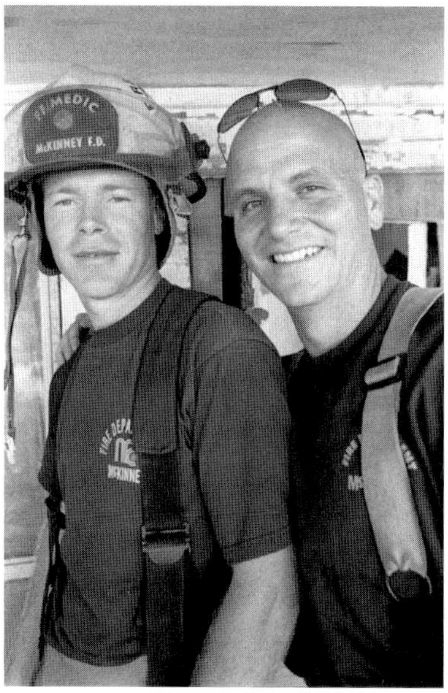
McKINNEY F.D.

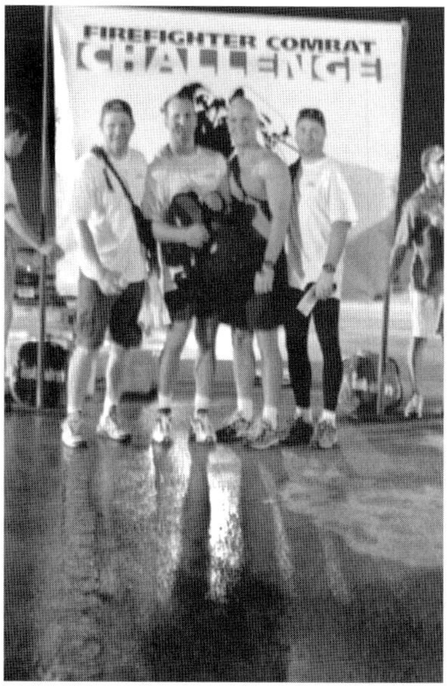
FIREFIGHTER COMBAT
CHALLENGE

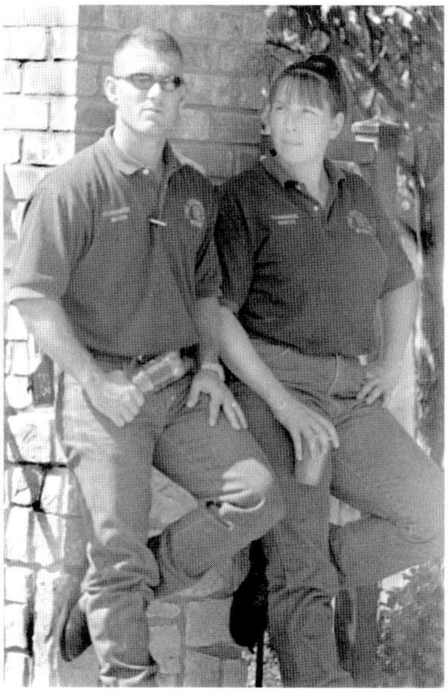

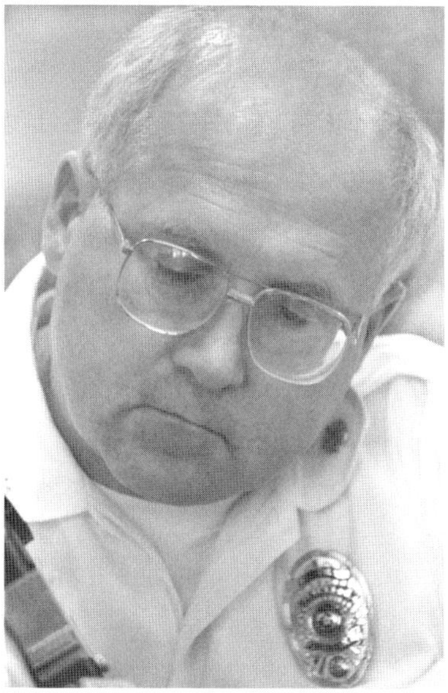

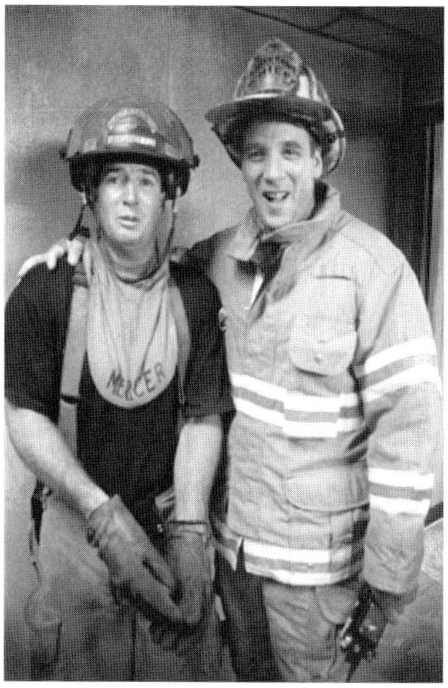
MERCER

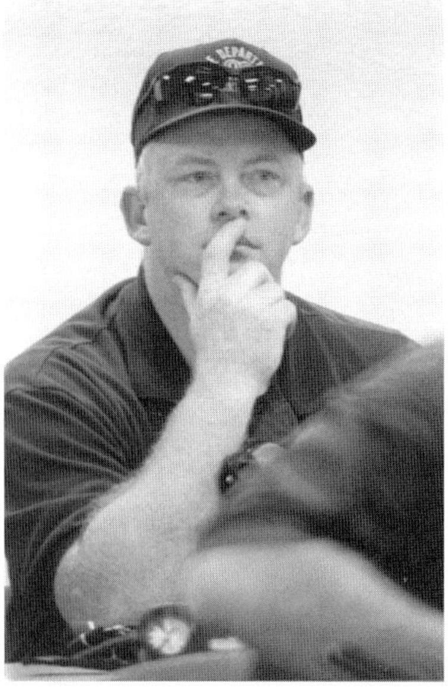

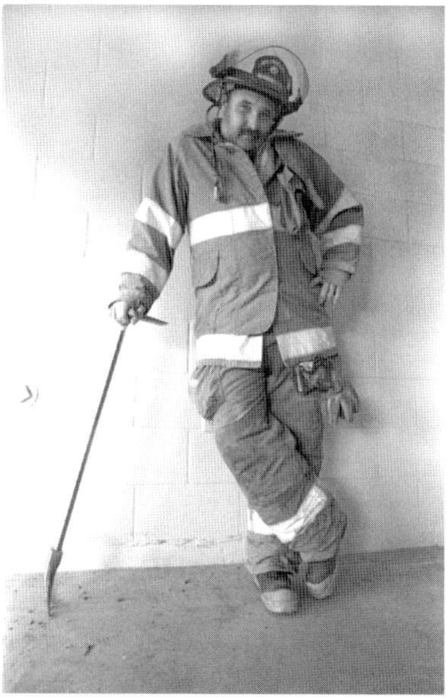

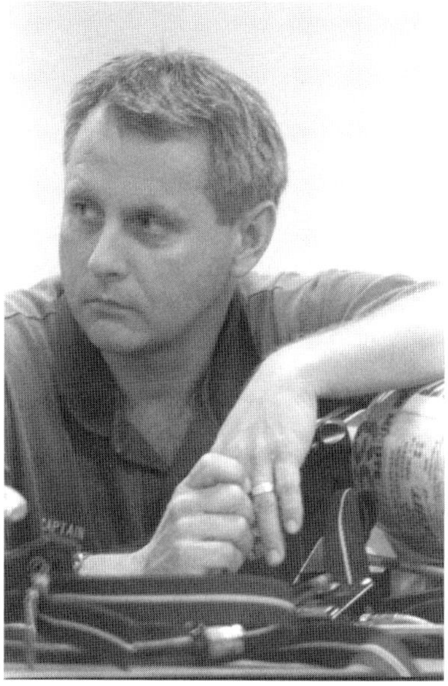

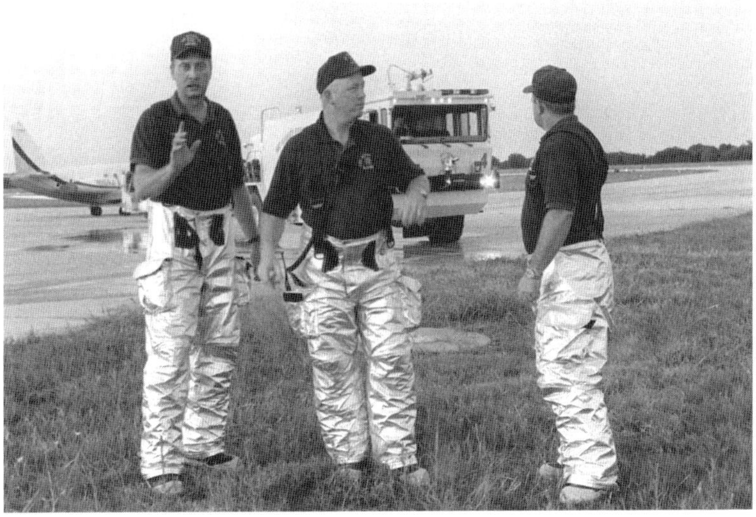

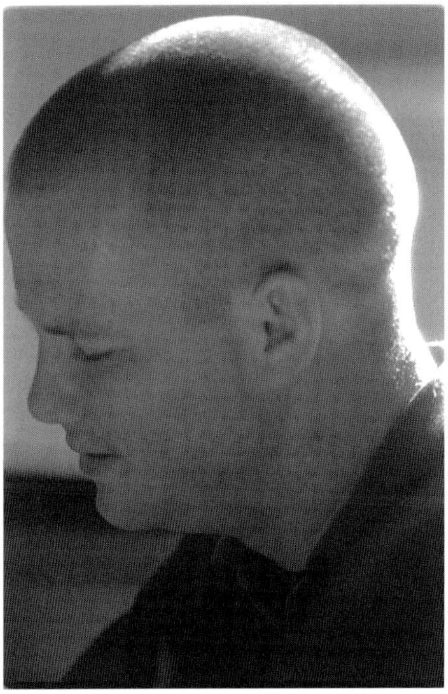

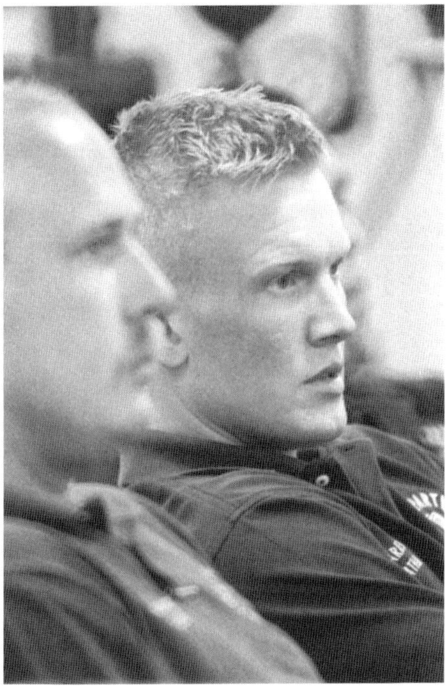

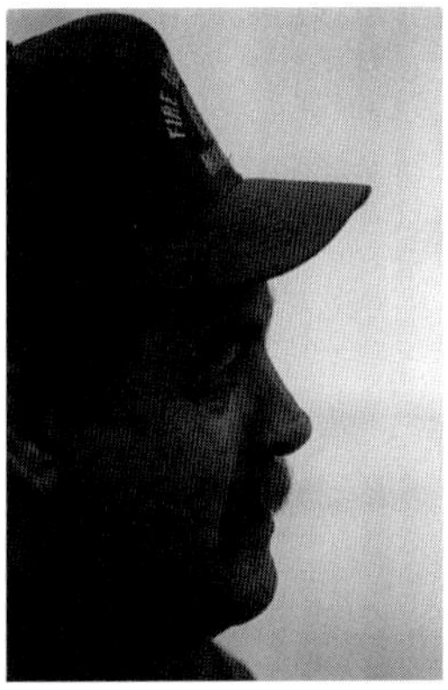

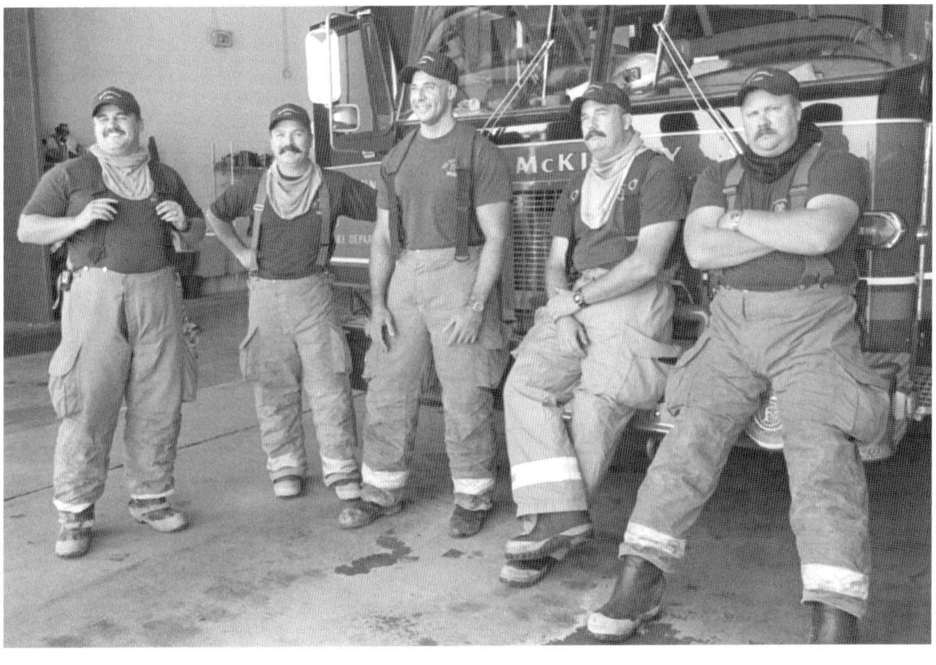
McKI

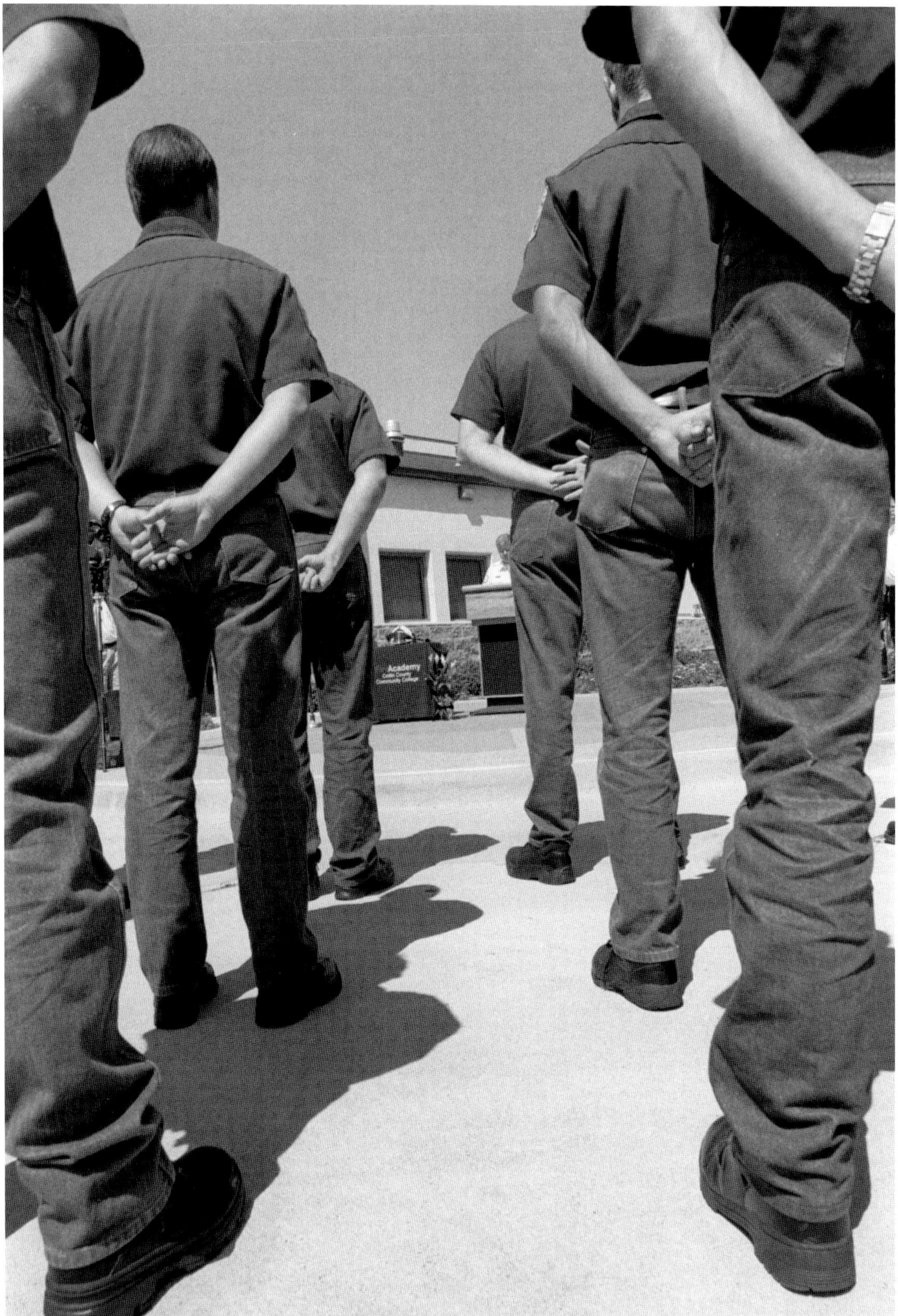
Academy

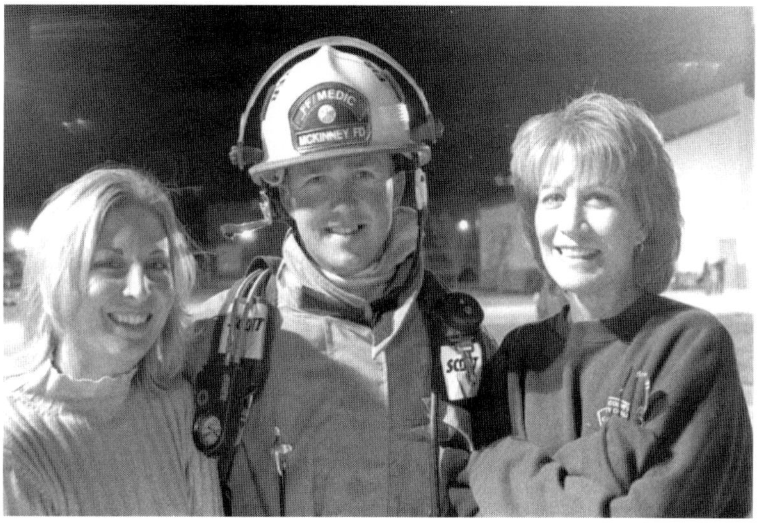
MCKINNEY FD

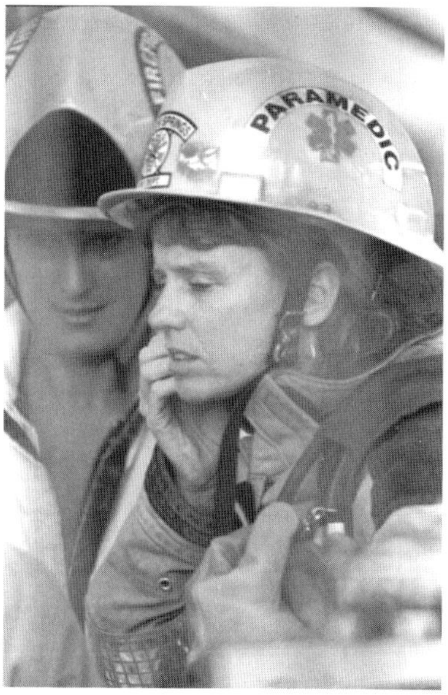
PARAMEDIC

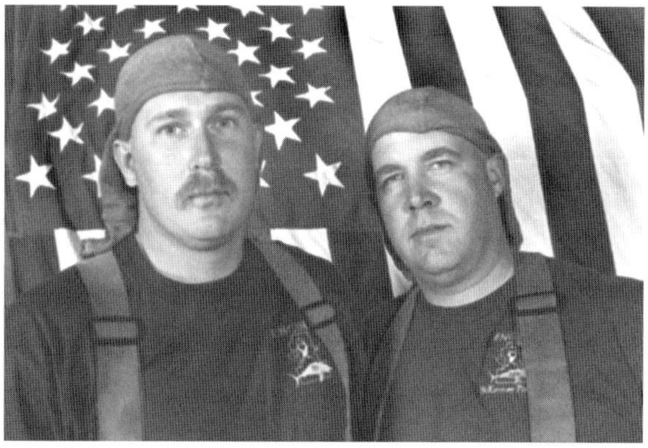

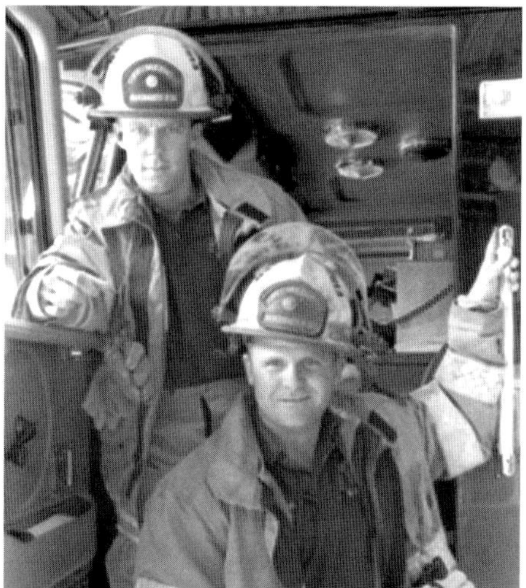

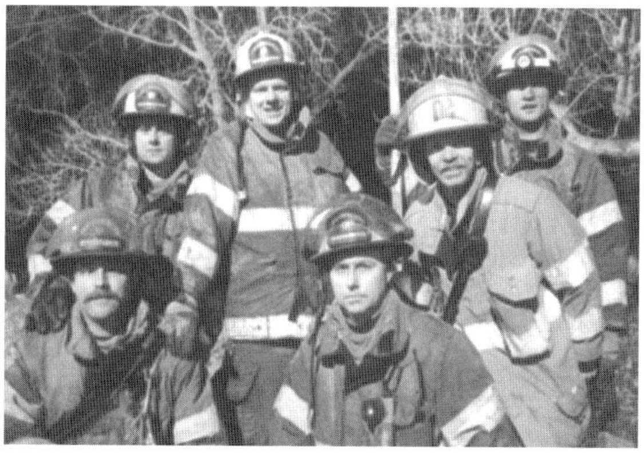

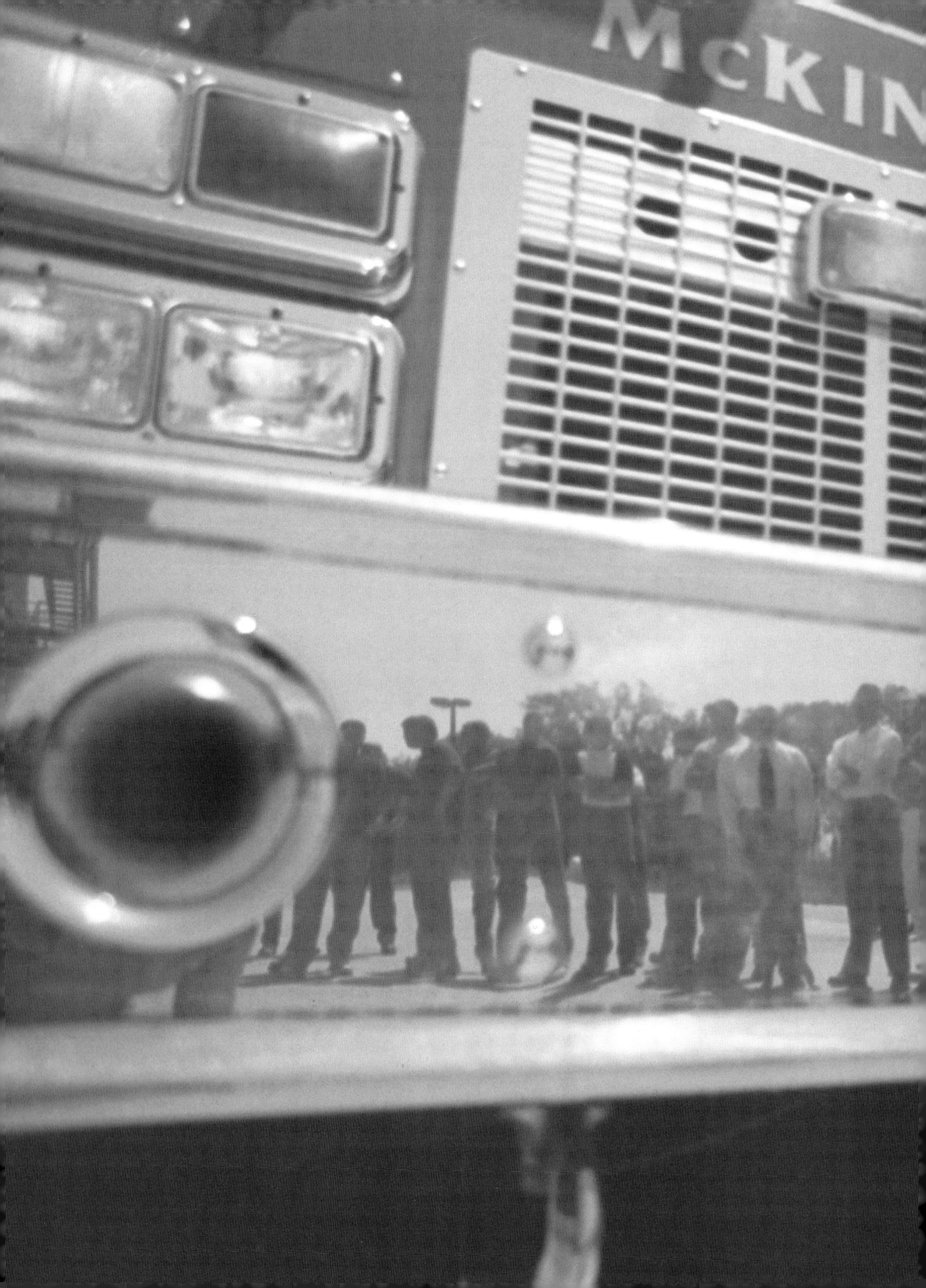
McKIN

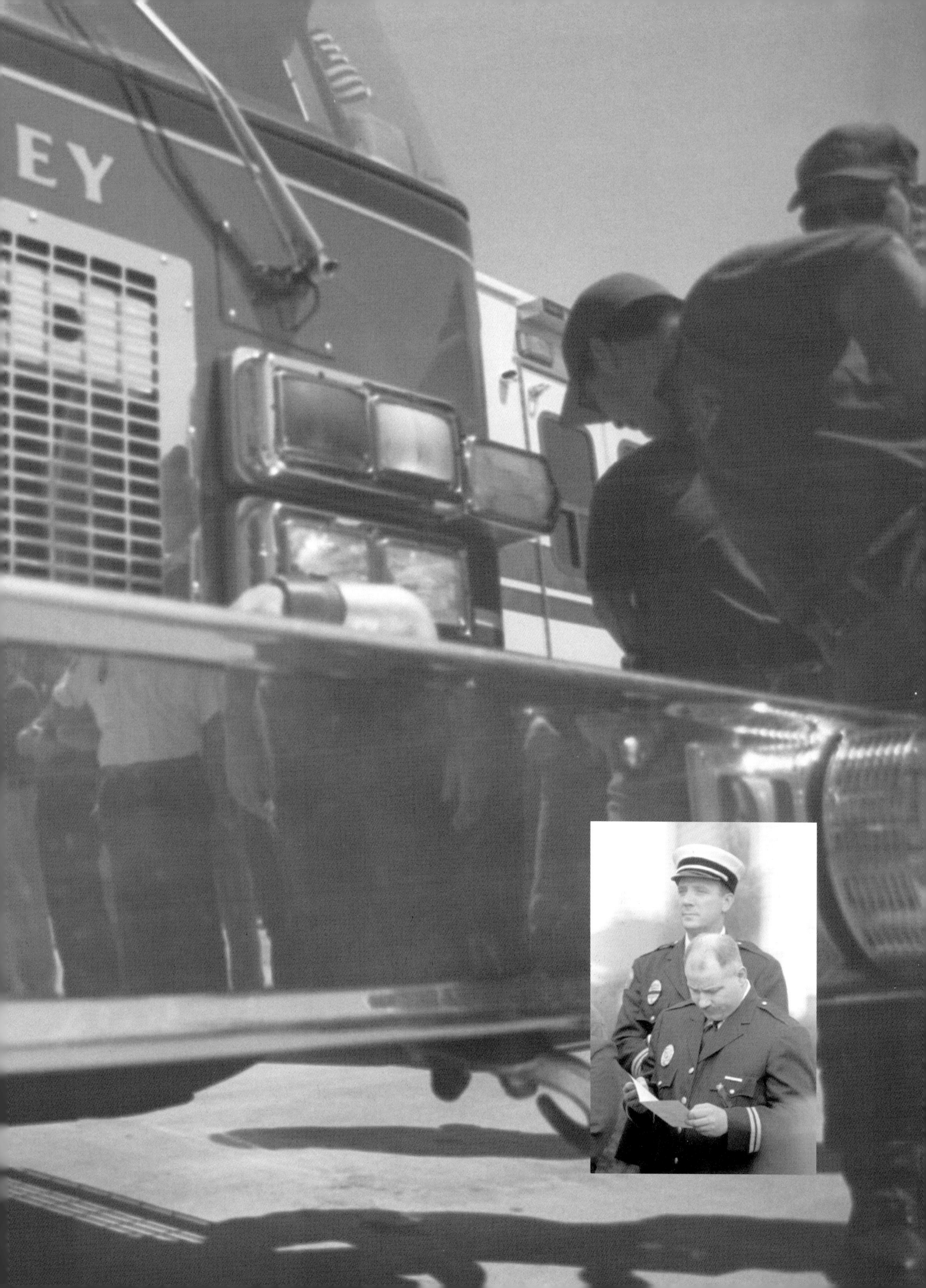
EY

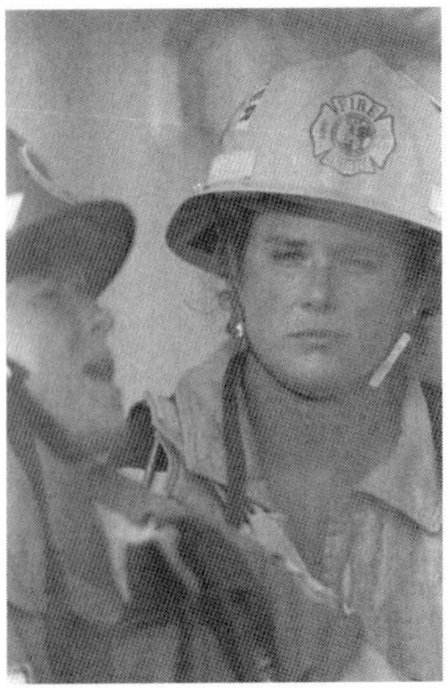

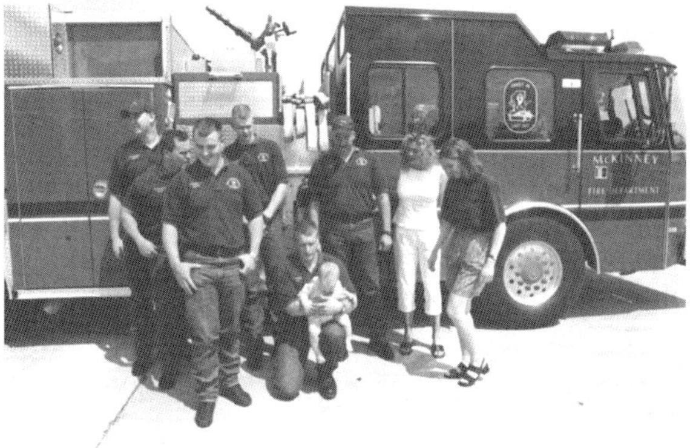
McKINNEY

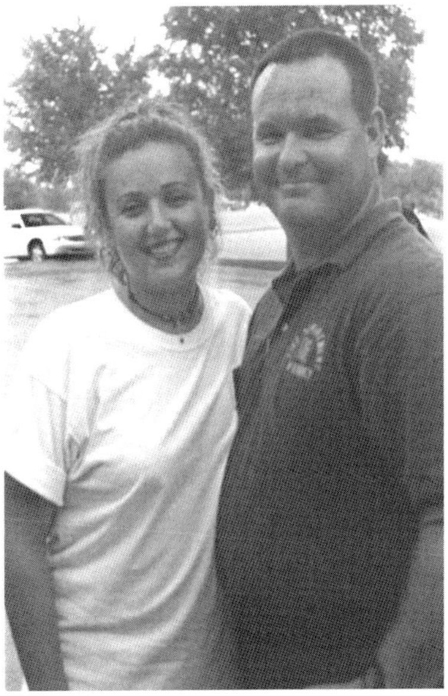

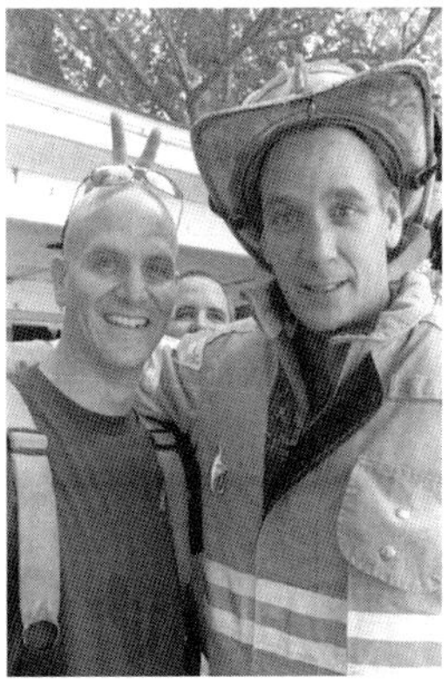

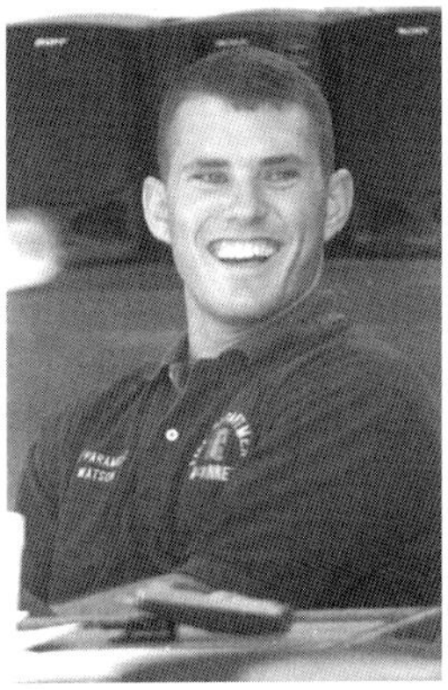

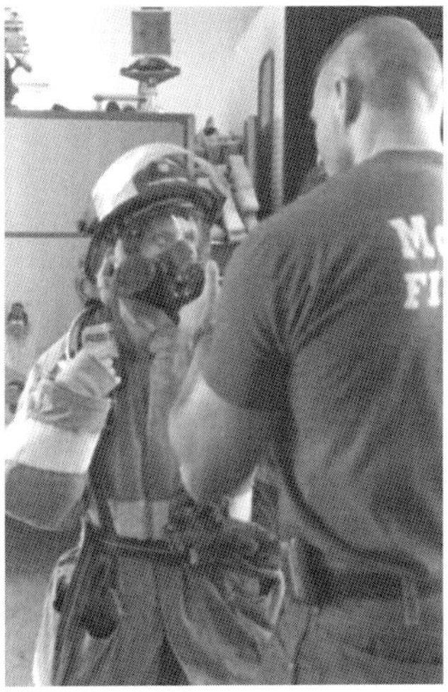

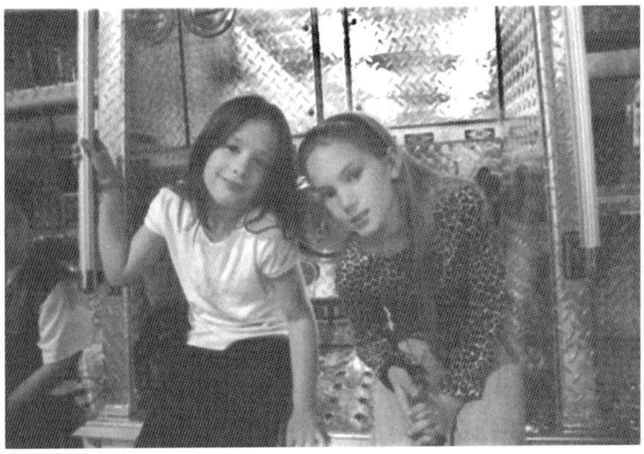

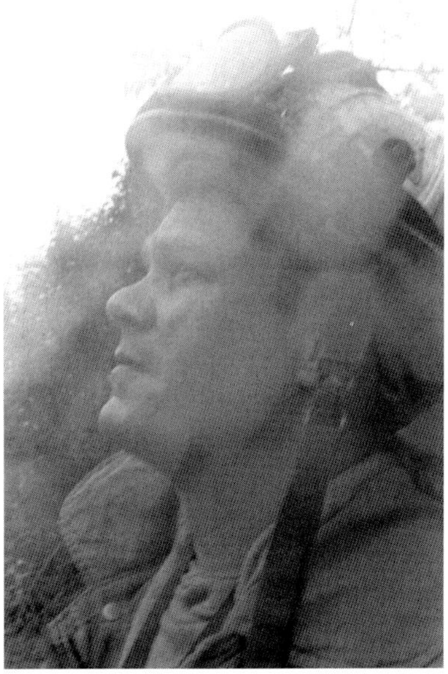

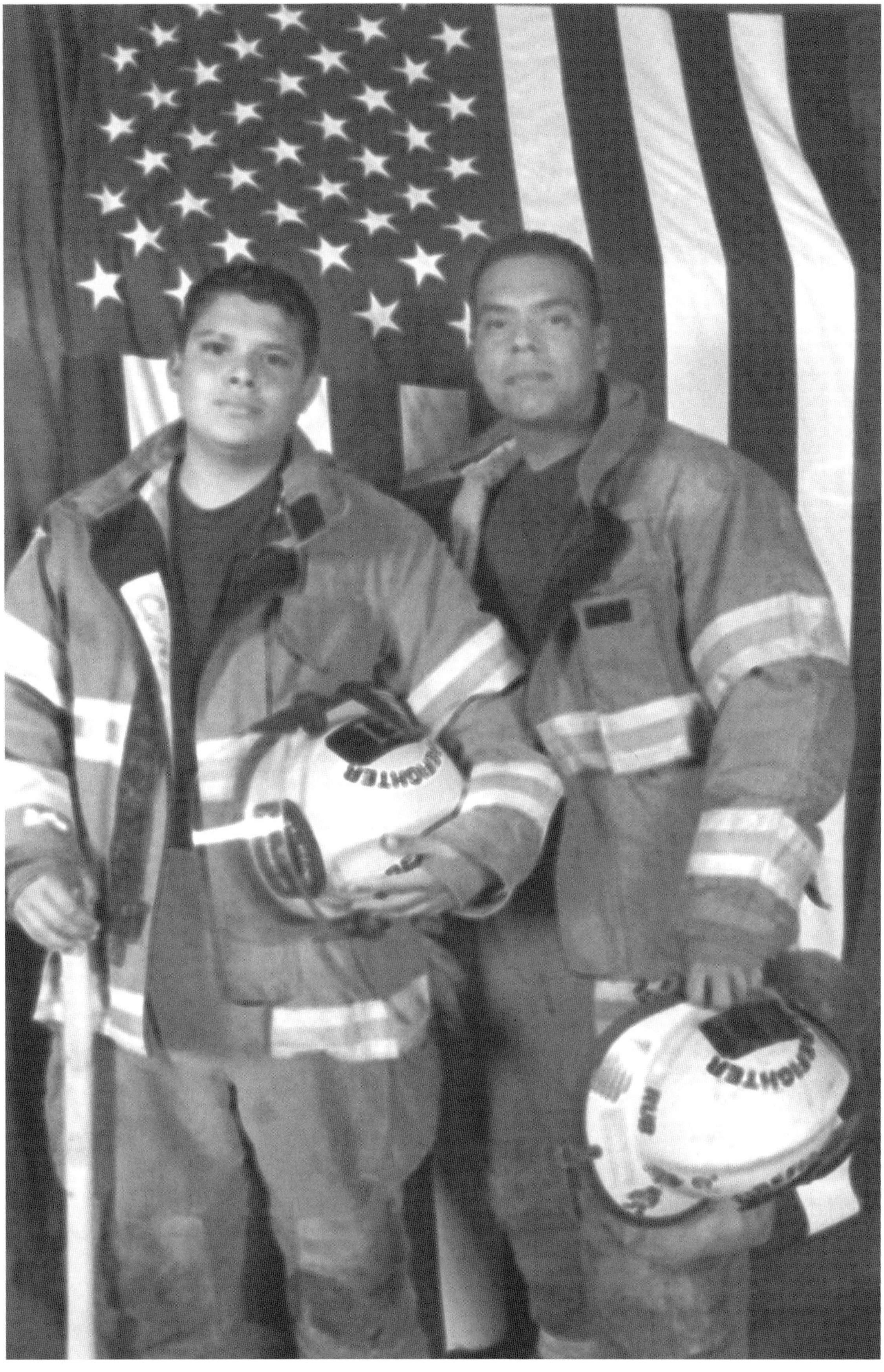

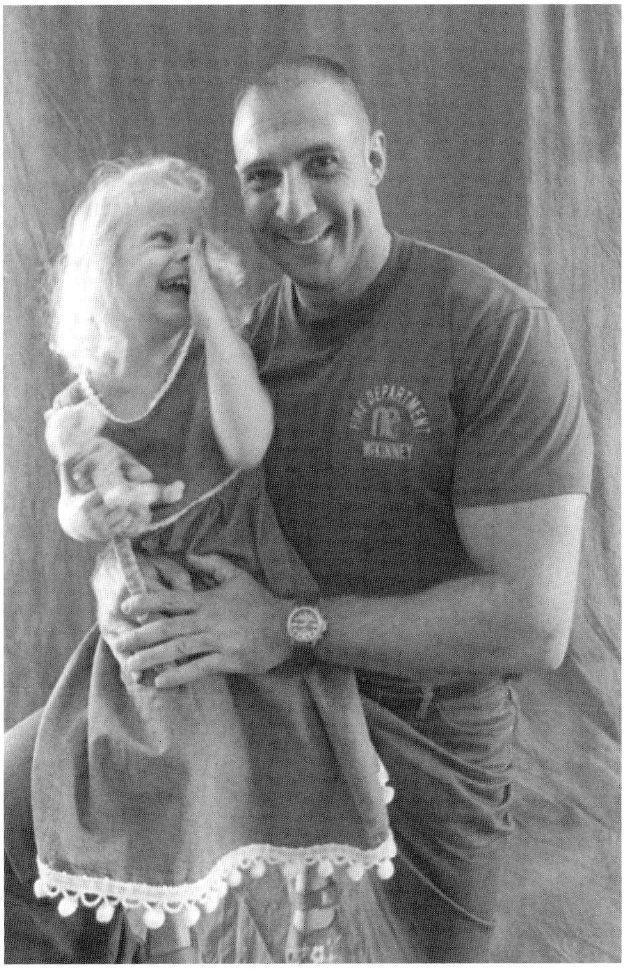
FIRE DEPARTMENT
McKINNEY

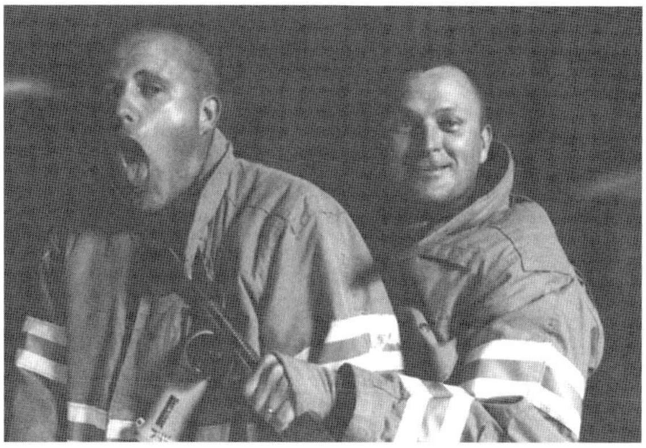

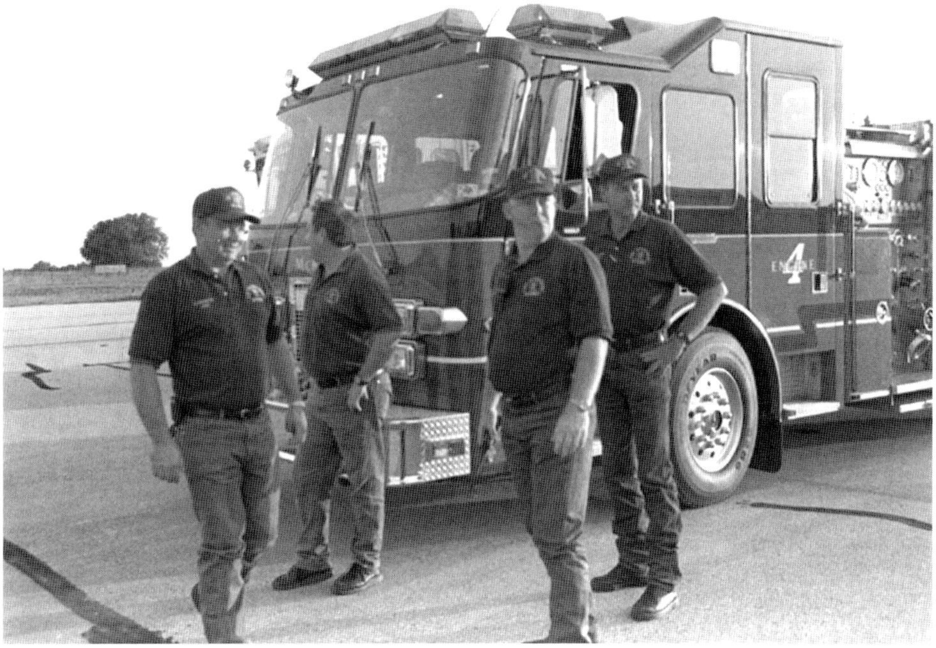

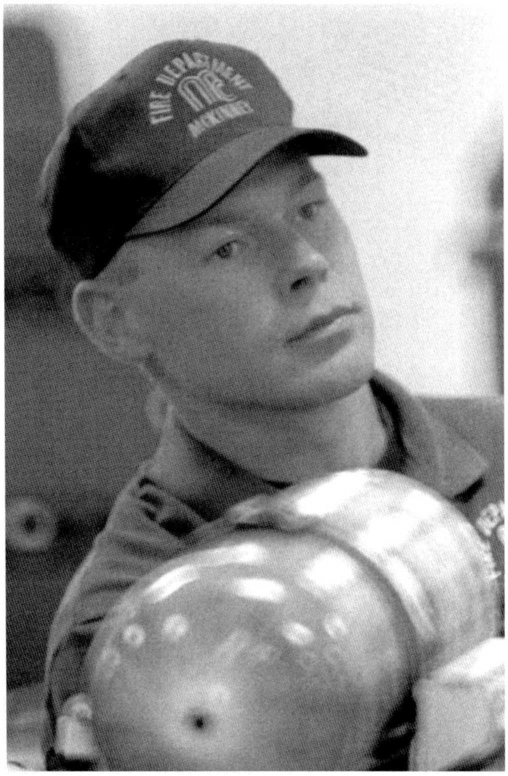

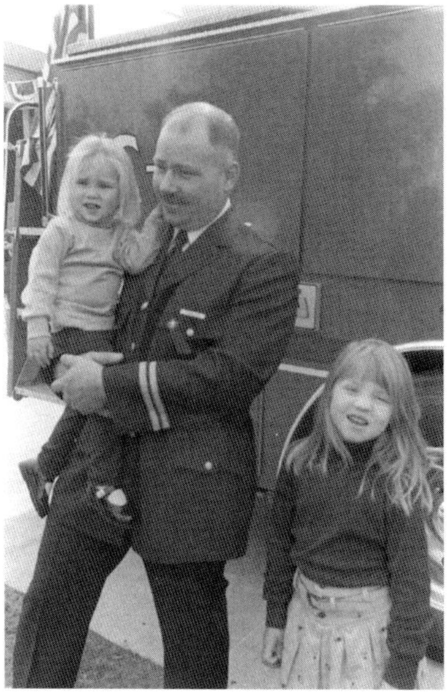

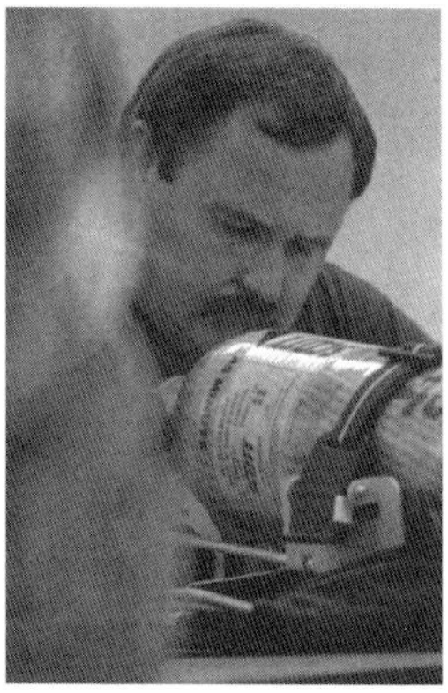

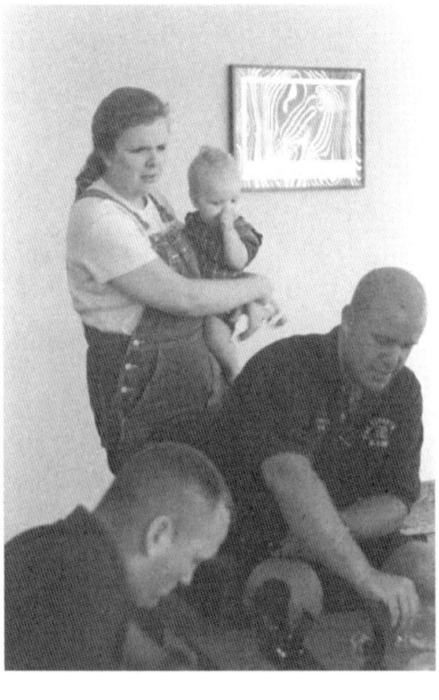

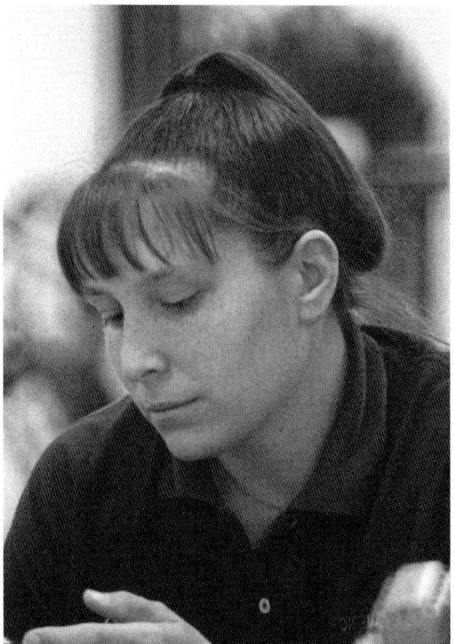

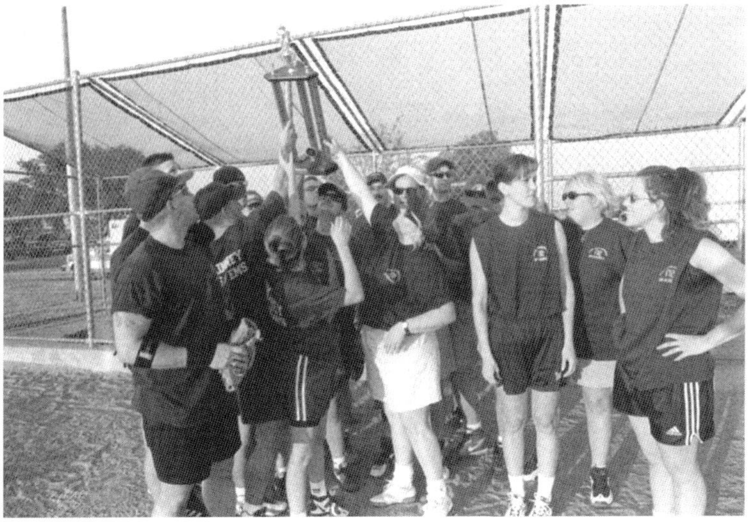

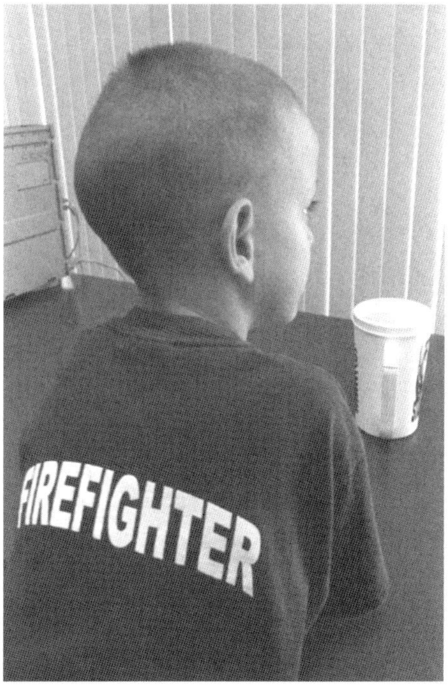
FIREFIGHTER

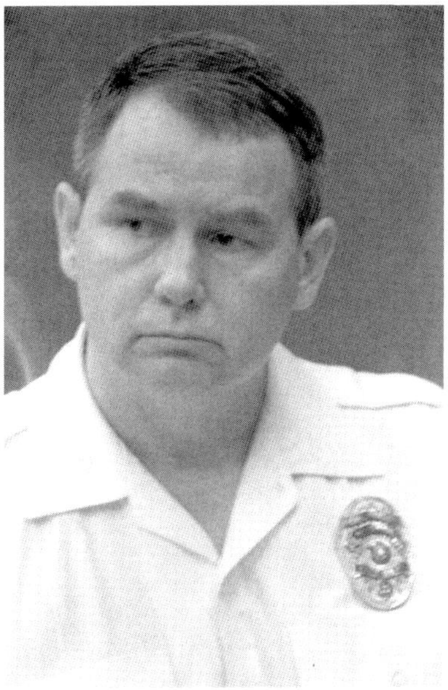

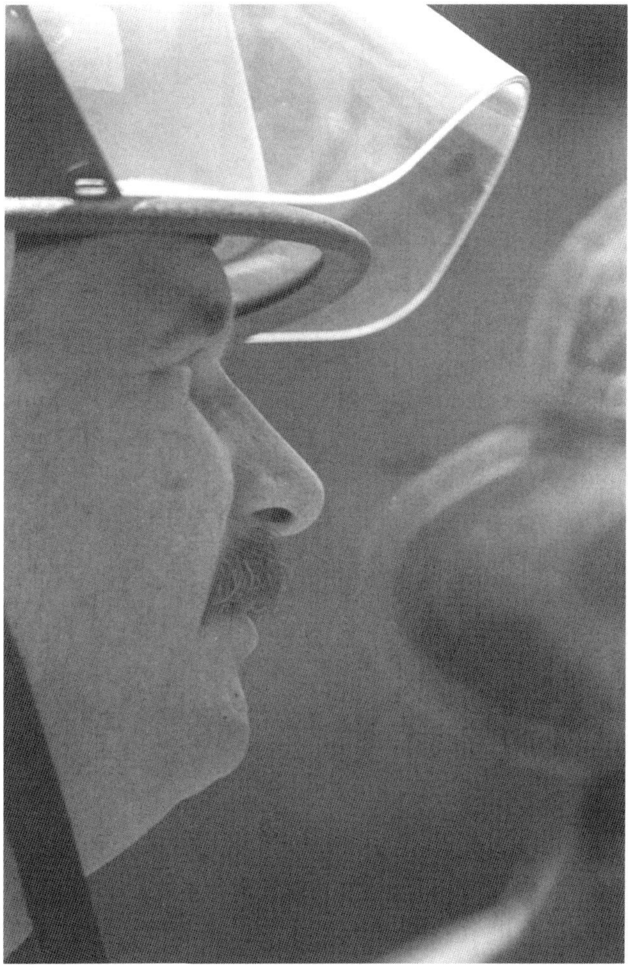

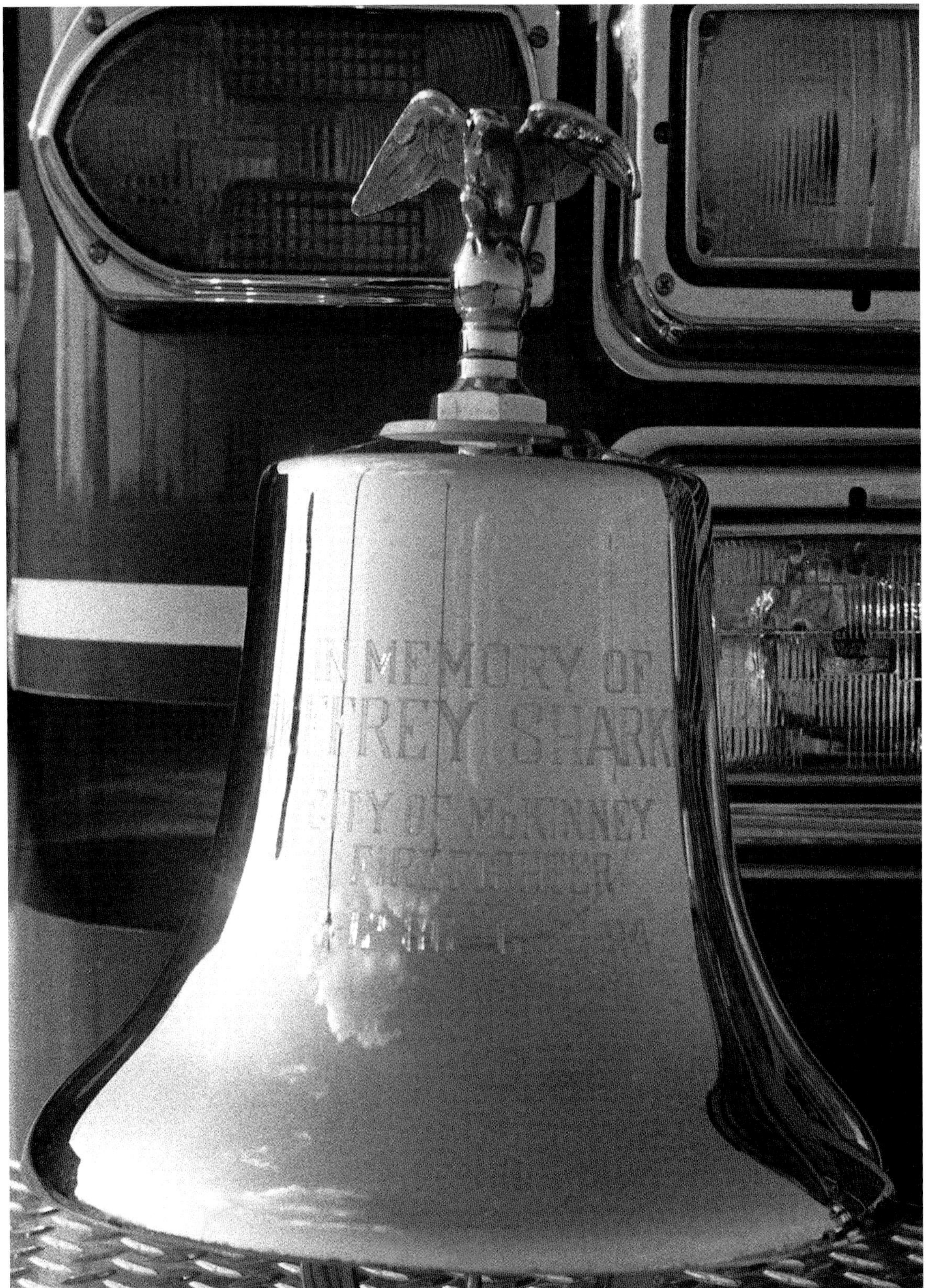
MEMORY OF

# notes

Most of the photographs in this book were taken impromptu at the scene or on location, not posed. As such, occasionally the quality of the image was affected by the circumstances of the situation. No flash or other artificial lighting was used, rather, only available light. I did attempt to present a natural and informal substance to the content and prints. By doing so, the images have a common realism that serves the subject and not that of studio or classic photographic art.

I am extremely thankful for both the physical and learning environments that encouraged and enabled me to conceive and later facilitate the realization of this book. Dr. Cary Israel, President of Collin County Community College District leads a great school with an educational program that excels by every measure. My experiences at CCCCD cultivated my progress as a photographer and inspired my venture to produce this book.

Additional copies of this book or archival prints, sized to your specifications, of any of the individual images may be obtained by contacting me at any of the following addresses or points of contact:

Pete Knudsen
pb publishing
a service of esense corporation (tx)
Box 9
Weston, Texas USA 75097-0009
972-382-2788 voice
972-382-3305 fax
writeus@esense corp.us

I will be pleased to respond to your inquiry regarding any aspect of the book, its content, circumstance or potential production of a similar volume. Thank you for your interest.

# acknowledgements

I want to formally and gratefully recognize the enthusiastic support and encouragement of my wonderful wife Andrea Bartosova Knudsen. Without her, nothing is possible. She has on several occasions, literally and figuratively, saved my life . This book is one more example.

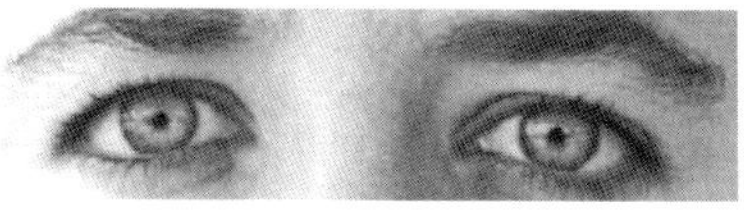

The project was also sustained by the invaluable guidance and contributing suggestions of:

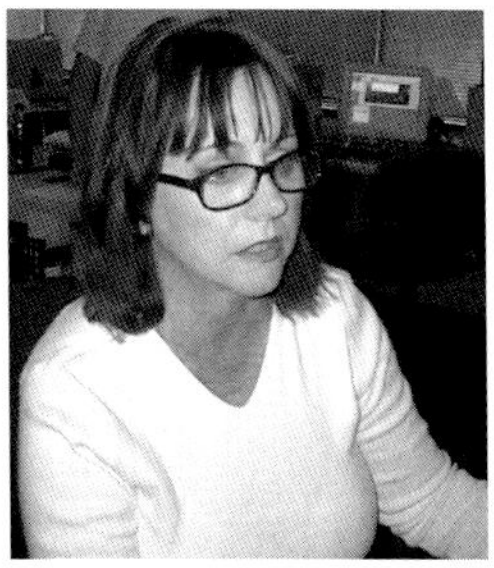

Victoria Clary

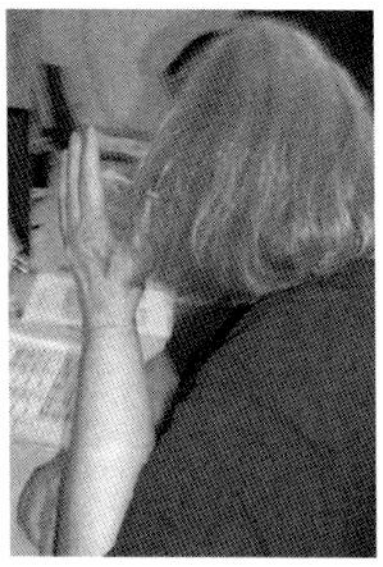

Marcia Barbour

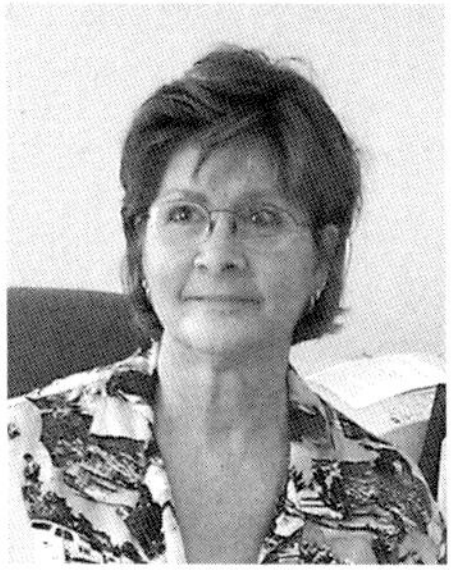

Nancy Eastham

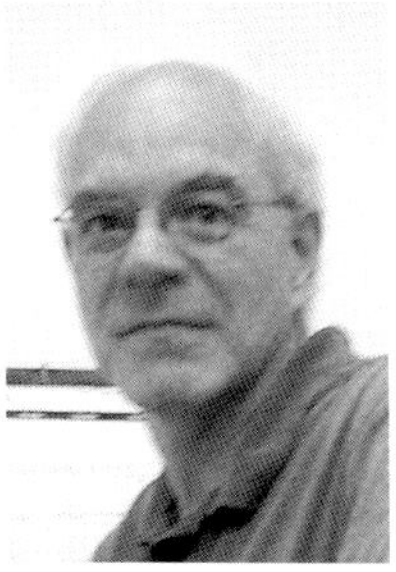

David Glosson

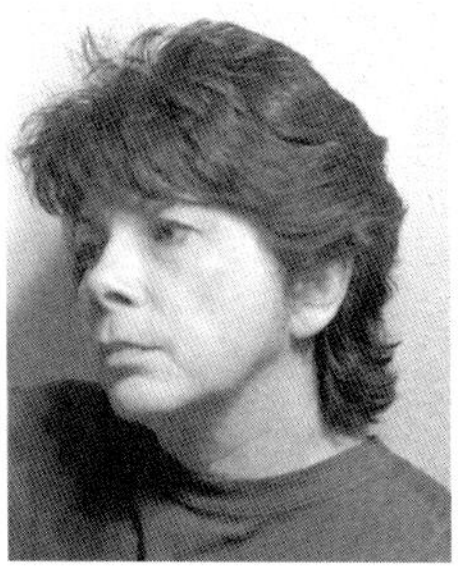

Gabrielle Pruitt

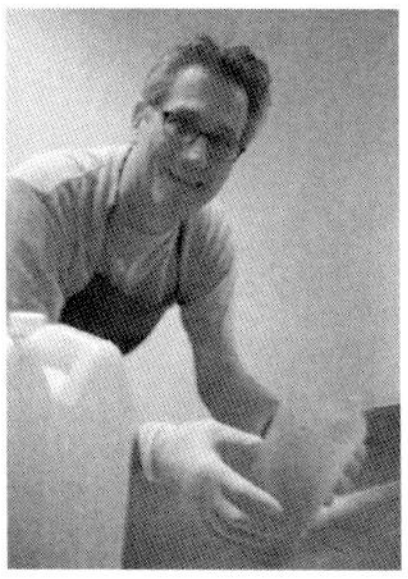

Byrd Williams

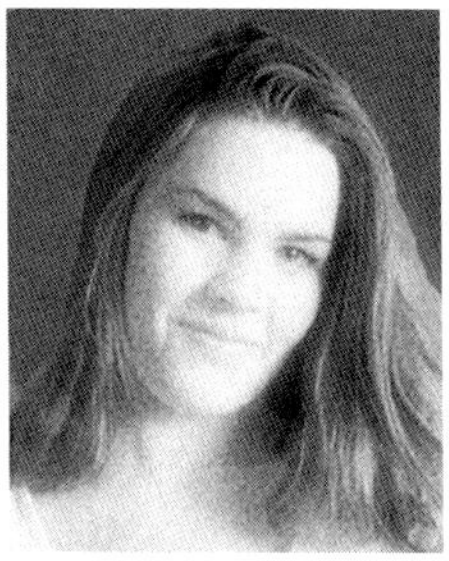

Rosalie Zentner-Wilson

*Thank you all for everything !*

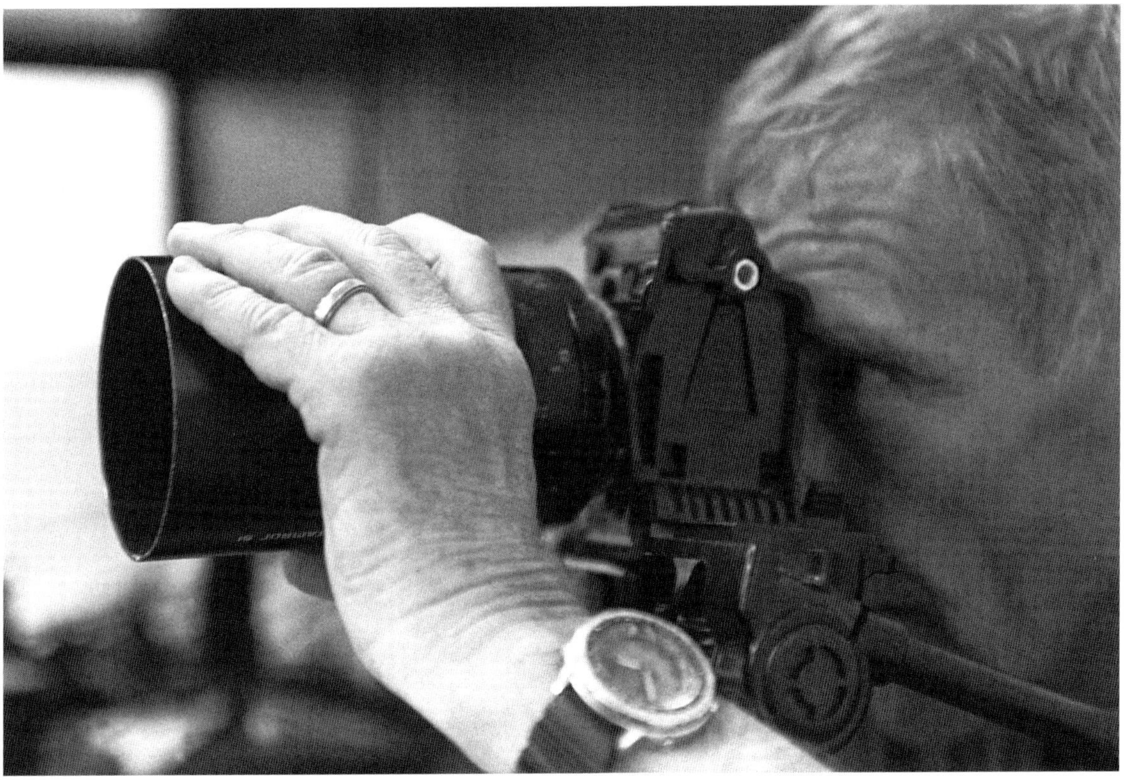

# colophon


| | |
|---|---|
| **Subject:** | Environment and activities of a community Fire Department |
| **Location:** | McKinney, Texas USA |
| **Time frame:** | June 2001 - April 2002 |
| **Cameras:** | 35mm:Nikon 8008s, Leica 1: # 12321; 4x5: Zone VI; Digital: D1X |
| **Lenses:** | Variety of Nikon, Leitz Elmar, Sigma, Calumet; fixed/variable |
| **Films:** | Ilford HP5 plus 400; Kodak TMax 3200 |
| **Developer:** | D-78 1:1 |
| **Scanner:** | Kodak RFS-2035 Pro V3.5 |
| **Hardware:** | Graphics: Apple G-4; Text: Dell xps 8600r |
| **Software:** | Graphics: Adobe Photoshop 6.0, Text: MS-Word 2000 |
| **File formats** | jpeg, pdf, tiff, doc |
| **Layout:** | Quark Express 4.1 |
| **Titles font:** | Impact 100 pt. |
| **Chapters font:** | Impact 80 pt. |
| **Text font:** | Garamond 12pt |
| **Printing:** | Thomson-Shore, Inc. Dexter, Mich. 48130-9701 |
| **Paper:** | 100lb Huron Gloss Enamel White, 526 ppi. |
| **Cover:** | IGC,Inc. Pearl Linen # 47240 ANSI "B" |
| **Jacket:** | 100lb Enamel UV |
| **Binding:** | Case, Smythe Stitch 16's; 98pt bbds, 80lb endsheets T-S Inc. |
| **Shipping standard:** | USPS |
| **Shipping air exp** | FedEx-US, USPS-Intn'l |